Enlighten, LLC
www.discovertruthwithin.com

Notice to Readers:

Original painting and cover art by Amanda Elton and graphic design by Mary Bitter.

Enlighten Presents

Emotional Healing
with Essential Oils

Manual I: Introduction

Daniel Macdonald

"The medical school of the future will not particularly interest itself in the ultimate results and products of disease, nor will it pay so much attention to actual physical lesions, or administer drugs and chemicals merely for the sake of palliating our symptoms, but knowing the true cause of sickness and aware that the obvious physical results are merely secondary it will concentrate its efforts upon bringing about the harmony between body, mind and soul which results in the relief and cure of disease"

"Amongst the types of remedies that will be used will be those obtained from the most beautiful plants and herbs to be found in the pharmacy of Nature, such as have been divinely enriched with healing powers for the mind and body of man"

—Dr. Edward Bach

Table of Contents

Section III: Appendices

Acknowledgements

The process of writing this manual has required the support of many people. I would first like to thank my patient wife, Julia. Thank you for encouraging me to publish this manual and for your continued patience as I labored over its creation. I want to acknowledge the loving support of my parents and family members.

I am also grateful to my partners in Enlighten: Amanda, Chuck, and Sarah for helping me bring this dream into reality. I have been inspired by your valiant hearts and your desire to share this material. Your tireless commitment to the vision has been incredible. I would also like to thank your families for sacrificing so much time with you as we worked on this project.

Additionally, I would also like to thank Amanda E. for the front and back cover art, Mary B. for design and formatting, and Katie B. and Jen K. for proofreading.

Finally, I would like to thank the earth for her abundant gifts, and God who inspires all truth and facilitates all healing.

Note from the Author

Dear Reader,

In the creation of this book I have used intuitive as well as alternative methods of research. I have felt humbled by the prospect of writing about the emotional and spiritual properties of the oils. It is like trying to summarize a dear friend in only a few sentences; how can you ever do them justice?

These oils are a true gift to mankind. They assist in healing both physically and spiritually. They support the mental and emotional fields. I believe that essential oils will play a major role in the healing of the planet and reversal of illness and disease. These oils have sustained me through long hours of writing. They have driven me forward, encouraging the completion of this first manual.

As far as I am aware, this book is the first of its kind. I have scavenged bookstores, aromatherapy volumes, and the web looking for this kind of information on oils. In my study, I have found that while oils are commonly referred to as "emotional healers," no one explained the specifics. I am not aware of any other resource on the market that describes the actual soul qualities of the oils.

I did not plan on writing this book for anyone else. Originally it was to be written for my personal use. I wanted to know what the oils did emotionally, so I set out on a journey to discover their properties. As I posted a few findings on my blog, people started responding with intense interest. Dozens of people ask each week when I'll publish more of my research. I do not want to keep people waiting any longer for this incredible information. I am excited to finally share this, the first volume in series of manuals on the emotional and spiritual properties of essential oils.

Sincerely,

Daniel Macdonald
December 2011
Alpine, Utah

Foreword

Though writing the forward for this book is a privilege, it is no small task. How do I consolidate decades of experience in order to share the scope through which I view this work? Regardless of the challenge, I hope to share a portion of my enthusiasm for the contents of these pages.

I have had the honor of working professionally in the field of holistic healing for over 16 years. As with most people, my personal journey began with a desire to improve my own health, which then spread to helping those around me. It fast became more than a hobby, and soon evolved into my mission and purpose.

During my time as a health practitioner and Holistic Health Coach, I had the honor of meeting Daniel Macdonald. We shared many moments of enlightenment, awareness and change. I knew then that he was an active observer of life, and willing to embrace the opportunity to examine life's lessons on a deeper level.

Years later, we reconnected with joint purpose and like-mindedness. I have worked with Daniel under a variety of circumstances and have rediscovered his wisdom and capacity. We both share a passion for teaching, inspiring and inviting all we come in contact with to experience healing. He has a divinely given ability to understand specific healing tools in both nature and application. As essential oils are one of Daniel's fortes, I challenged him to capture his passion and expound on his discoveries and research in a resource that could be shared. I have loved observing Daniel's dedication to the project and his demand for quality. He patiently and painstakingly gathered, organized, and refined, then gathered more, and refined more until he could offer a quality product. I am immensely grateful to Daniel for his determination to dig, discover, delve and then divulge his knowledge of the oils contained in these pages.

I've had the opportunity to use Daniel's preliminary findings prior to the release of this work, and have found them to be incredibly accurate. As I utilized Daniel's research, I have shared many moments of pure awareness with loved ones and strangers alike. Through much experience and application, I can confidently state that Daniel's descriptions of each oil have blessed many lives with a new degree of consciousness. This book offers a level of insight that is amazing. Many individuals have wondered how the oils could so precisely "peg" their emotional and spiritual states.

It is with excitement and confidence that I invite you to discover for yourself the wisdom of this work. Kallie's story is but one of the incredible examples of healing that essential oils can bring.

Enjoy the enlightenment!

Laura Jacobs

Laura has been a practitioner in the health and wellness industry for 16 years, serving over 15,000 clients. She is an herbalist and aromatherapist, and practices iridology, kinesiology, nutrition and life coaching. Laura is also a Blue Diamond with dōTERRA International.

Section I

Healing
with Essential Oils

Kallie's Story

The following true story, written by Kallie's mother, perfectly embodies the steps involved in emotional healing- from the time of trauma, through the healing crisis, and on to wholeness. It beautifully illustrates how the use of essential oils facilitates healing, physically, emotionally and spiritually. We sincerely thank Kallie and her family for allowing this story to be included in this book.

When my daughter Kallie was two years old, she accidentally pulled a crock-pot full of boiling meat down onto herself, severely burning her face and torso. Second and third degree burns covered a third of her body. For a month Kallie recuperated in a special burn unit where she received heavy narcotics along with other medications to help numb the intense pain that accompanies such severe burns. Two surgeries were necessary to place skin grafts on her face, neck and shoulders. When Kallie finally came home, she had to wear a plastic mask on her face and a tight fitting body suit for six months to keep the skin grafts from warping.

As her mother, it was horrifying to see my child suffer so much pain. I felt helpless. But Kallie is a very strong girl who tried her best to adapt to the excruciating medical procedures, such as having the dead skin scrubbed from the burned area or working through physical therapy. During the many times when the pain and trauma was too much for little Kallie, she would mentally leave us. I could see it in her hollow eyes. The first time I saw this was when the initial burn happened. In those few seconds right after the hot liquid touched her precious skin, she wasn't there. Due to the combination of heavy narcotics and unbearable procedures, she was physically and emotionally numb or just plain absent during most of the month that she was hospitalized. After we got home, it took a while to get back to regular life. Kallie was just so fragile and delicate. I tried my absolute best to physically and emotionally recover her and our family from this event, but it was quite a challenge.

The months and years went by, and I started to notice that Kallie was extremely numb to pain. She is a very active, adventurous girl and would have quite a few falls and injuries just like any other child, but she would rarely acknowledge that it hurt her. Sometimes it was disturbing. I remember one visit to the doctor for her regular vaccines. Kallie was lying down on the table and the two nurses poked both her legs two times each. I was watching her face, and there was absolutely no physical or emotional reaction whatsoever. She was unfeeling. She would often get nasty gashes or scrapes, and I wouldn't even know about it until later when I would give her a bath or change her clothes. I would ask her where she got hurt, and a lot of times she wouldn't even remember. She was also very self-conscious of the physical changes the burn had caused. When Kallie began school, she would try to hide her scars by covering them with her hair or coat or by walking with her face pointed towards the wall and away from onlookers.

I never pushed her to talk about it or do anything that was uncomfortable for her, but I gently tried to give her opportunities to share her thoughts and feelings. When Kallie was about five and a half, she started to forget what happened. She knew that something big occurred a long time ago, but she couldn't remember the details. Sometimes there was a trigger that sparked her memory, like the word "burn," or a fire, or even a bath. Then with fear and confusion in her eyes she would start asking, "What happened to me, Mom?" Around this time, I was introduced to essential oils. As my mother and I learned about the oils and their benefits, we thought of Kallie. Helichrysum and Vetiver seemed like the perfect fit, and we began treatment. I was so excited in the beginning, mostly thinking of the potential physical healing and largely unaware of the emotionally benefits. Kallie was full of faith. She immediately said, "I know it's gonna make my burn melt away Mom!" I had no idea what was coming.

After only a few days of using the oils, Kallie started to act differently. The first thing I noticed was that she started to complain of physical pain for which we could find no reasonable explanation. Every time she would get the smallest cut or bruise, she would have major anxiety about it—very opposite from her recent tough and "numb-to-pain" reactions. She would cry for hours about a tiny cut or sliver and would say through tears, "Is it ever gonna go away?" Kallie spent a large portion of the day worrying about the smallest things. It was almost impossible to convince her to take a bath. She became extremely picky about the clothes she wore. If clothing touched her "wrong" or was at all tight, she wouldn't wear it. Any mention of her being burned or even the word "burn" would cause extreme fear. Anxiety attacks surfaced. Sometimes she would randomly sit on my lap and just cry. I would cry too.

I finally realized Kallie was going through a healing crisis brought on by the oils. It made perfect sense. Every odd thing that she was doing directly correlated to the burn or to her experience in the hospital. With the help of essential oils, her body was expelling or ejecting all of the pain and hidden emotions that were buried for so long.

We guessed that the healing would probably last for the same amount of time she had stayed in the hospital. This was exactly right. It lasted a month. I tried my best to validate what she was feeling and to help her as much as I could during this time. I learned that if I missed a day of putting on her oils, it was a bad day for her and the rest of the household! So, I kept up with it, and the results were phenomenal.

After this difficult month I began to notice that words which had previously triggered a negative reaction from Kallie did not seem to bother her. She had a totally new and positive perspective. I could see plain as day that she was no longer coming from a place of fear. Instead of being self-conscious or shy, she was secure, strong and confident—a totally different Kallie.

As her mom, I can see without a doubt that these essential oils gave her such a beautiful new outlook on herself and her past traumatic experience. On the morning of Kallie's seventh birthday, I was telling her about the day she was born, and she said, "I don't remember that, Mom, but I do remember when I was burned." I carefully asked, "What do you feel when you remember it?" She replied in her bubbly, secure voice, "Let me spell it for you mom: OK!" Words cannot express how very grateful I am that my little Kallie could heal emotionally.

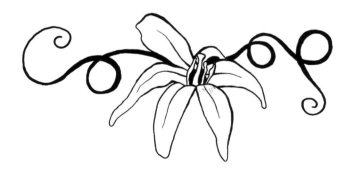

Healing Emotions
with Essential Oils

As was just illustrated in Kallie's story, essential oils play a powerful role in emotional healing. They lead us by the hand as we courageously face our emotional issues. Kallie is not the only one with repressed emotional trauma. We all hold unresolved feelings of pain and hurt which need to be brought to the surface for transformation and healing.

Essential Oils: Five Stages of Healing

Essential oils support healing in five stages. They strengthen us during each stage and prepare us for the next level of healing. For example, as we regain our physical health, we are invited to enter the emotional realm.

In this manual we will briefly explore stage one and mainly focus on defining stage two: the emotional stage. While we briefly touch on the third through fifth stages throughout this manual, they are largely topics for another book.

The Five Stages are:

1. Essential oils assist in healing the physical body

2. Essential oils assist in healing the heart

3. Essential oils assist in releasing limiting beliefs

4. Essential oils increase spiritual awareness and connection

5. Essential oils inspire the fulfillment of our life's purpose

Stage One: Healing the Physical Body

Essential oils are powerful physical healers. They assist the body in fighting unfriendly micro-organisms, purifying organs and glands, and balancing body functions. Some essential oils are considered to be 40 to 60 times more potent than herbs. Oils range from being anti-bacterial, to anti-viral, and anti-inflammatory in nature. Essential oils rapidly heal the physical body, raise the body's vibration and balance the systems of the body.

Stage Two: Healing the Heart

As the oils secure our physical health, they provide us with the energy needed to penetrate the heart and enter the emotional realm. Essential oils raise the vibration of the physical body. As the body lives in higher vibrations, lower energies (suppressed emotions) become unbearable. These feelings want to release. Stagnant anger, sadness, grief, judgment and low self-worth cannot exist in the environment of balance and peace, which essential oils help to create.

Healing is experienced as old feelings surface and release. Sometimes this experience is confused with regression. People may perceive they are going backwards or that the essential oils are not working. In reality, the oils are working. They are working to permanently heal emotional issues by supporting individuals through their healing crises.
We are so used to symptomatic healing that we have been conditioned to view healing as the immediate cessation of all physical and emotional pain.

Principles of Healing: Release and Replace

It is important to understand that healing is a process. The process can be separated into two main principles: release and replace.

We must release trapped negative emotions before we can receive positive feelings. The old must go to make space for the new. We often want to skip this step, but it is a necessary one. We must be willing to experience the cleansing if we truly desire healing. Resisting the cleansing process makes healing more painful. We must surrender to the experience so that we may continue on the path of healing. The more we let go and trust, the more enjoyable this healing process can be.

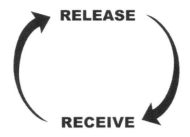

Essential Oils Don't Do Our Emotional Work for Us

Essential oils assist individuals in taking an honest look within. They foster the right environment for healing, but they will not do the work for us. In gardening, it is a common experience to pull the weeds while leaving the roots. This is particularly true for hard and rocky soils. To ensure we uproot the whole plant, we can add water to the soil, which allows the entire weed to be removed. Similarly, essential oils prepare our emotional soil so that weeds may be removed with greater ease. However, they do not do the weeding for us. If one neglects to do the work of pulling their weeds, they have simply watered the problem. On the other hand, those who combine essential oils with emotional work reap the fruit of their labor.

Tools for Emotional Work

You may be wondering, "How do I begin my emotional work?" Enlighten strives to provide quality products and services to assist people in their healing. In addition, we propose that individuals may begin their emotional work with a few introductory practices. We suggest meditation, journaling and personal inventory to facilitate the healing process.

We invite everyone to embark on their own healing path. We believe this book will greatly assist you and your family. We hope you will consider Enlighten an asset on your healing journey.

A Word on Quality

Three Categories of Essential Oils:

1. Aromatic Essential Oils
2. Therapeutic Grade Essential Oils
3. Certified Pure Therapeutic Grade (CPTG®) Essential Oils

The first category applies to many oils marketed for their scent and aromatic purposes. These essential oils are widely available in health food stores everywhere. It is important to know that these essential oils are not therapeutic grade and should not be used topically or internally, as they are not for medicinal use. These oils are usually synthetic and therefore harmful to the body. They have no therapeutic value whatsoever.

The Second category of essential oils is therapeutic grade. Many companies fall into this category. The intent of these companies is to provide quality essential oils that can be used for healing. These oils are for topical use. Great care should be taken when purchasing these oils, as they are often diluted with synthetic chemical or other additives.

The third category of essential oils is Certified Pure Therapeutic Grade (CPTG®). This label means they are safe not only for topical application, but also for internal use. CPTG® oils are tested at independent laboratories to certify their purity and composition. Because of the rigorous testing involved, CPTG® essential oils are a rare commodity. Never use any oil internally that is not certified as safe for dietary consumption by the FDA. dōTERRA is currently the only company which has met the CPTG® standard for quality and purity. This is why we have chosen dōTERRA essential oils for this manual. Only the highest quality oils can be used for physical, emotional and spiritual healing.

How to Use This Manual

Oil Descriptions

The main body of the manual is broken down into individual descriptions of the oils. The single oils are listed first, the oil blends next. You may read the individual oil or blend descriptions to determine which essential oil would be best suited for your emotional needs.

Usage Guide

Following the oil descriptions are special appendix topics including the usage guide. In the usage guide you may search for specific emotional states or imbalances and find their recommended oil.

Companion to Modern Essentials

This manual may also be used as a companion to *Modern Essentials*. After finding the recommended oils for your physical condition, cross-reference *Emotional Healing with Essential Oils*. As you read the oil descriptions, choose the oil(s) that match your emotional state as well as your physical condition.

Muscle Test

If you are familiar with muscle testing, you may reference *Application Though Muscle Testing* in the appendix.

Section II

Oil Descriptions

SINGLE OILS

Basil

The Oil of Renewal

The symptoms of adrenal exhaustion help us to understand the main moods that are treated with Basil, primarily: overwhelm, fatigue, low energy and the inability to cope with life's stressors. The smell of Basil oil brings strength to the heart and relaxation to the mind. This oil is also excellent for states of nervousness, anxiety and depression.

Basil oil is helpful for those who are under a great deal of mental strain. It brings rejuvenation of vital forces after long periods of burnout and exhaustion. Basil oil helps heal the adrenals and restore the body to its natural rhythms of sleep, activity and rest.

Basil oil is also helpful for addiction recovery. It gives hope and optimism to the tired soul. In short, Basil is indicated for those who are weary in mind and body and for those in need of strength and renewal.

Suggested Uses: Place 3-5 drops on bottom of feet morning and night. Inhale regularly throughout the day.

Emotions Addressed: Anxious, Weary, Overwhelmed, Tired, Drained, Exhausted, Addicted

Bergamot

The Oil of Self-Acceptance

Bergamot relieves feelings of despair, self-judgment and low self-esteem. It supports the individual in need of self-acceptance and self-love. Bergamot invites individuals to see life with more optimism.

Bergamot has a cleansing affect on stagnant feelings and limiting belief systems. Because of individuals' core beliefs of being "bad," "unlovable" and "not good enough," they seek to hide behind a façade of cheerfulness. They may fear revealing their true thoughts and feelings. Bergamot's powerful cleansing properties generate movement in the energy system, which in turn brings hope.

In this way, Bergamot is a wonderful anti-depressant. It awakens the soul to hope and offers courage to share the inner-self. Re-igniting optimism and confidence in the self, it imparts true self-acceptance. Bergamot teaches us to let go of self-judgment by learning to love ourselves unconditionally.

Suggested Uses: Place a drop under tongue. Place 2-3 drops over solar plexus. Inhale regularly throughout the day.

Emotions Addressed: Despair, Low self-esteem, Self-Judgment, Unlovable

Birch

The Oil of Support

Birch offers support to the unsupported. When a person is feeling attacked or unsupported by family or friends, Birch offers courage to move forward alone. Learning to be flexible is important, but so is gaining a strong backbone. Birch offers support to the weak-willed so that they may stand tall and firm in what they believe.

Birch helps us to feel our roots, specifically our connection to family and ancestors. Birch is a tree that stands tall and firm and it offers us support in doing the same. It assists us in overcoming negative generational patterns, especially in situations where one is at risk of being rejected if they choose a different way. It lends it's spirit of endurance to help us face trials of adversity so that we may weather any storm with the strength and conviction of a tree.

Birch teaches us that there is more to life than pain, and that with the right support and the right grounding, we too can be held up and sustained by Divine grace.

Suggested Uses: Place 1-3 drops along the spine or on the bottom of the feet. Inhale throughout the day.

Emotions Addressed: Unsupported, Alienated, Fear, Weak-Willed

Cassia

The Oil of Self-Assurance

Cassia brings gladness and courage to the heart and soul. It is a wonderful remedy for the shy and timid. It helps those who hold back and try to hide. When a person avoids being the center of attention, Cassia can restore their confidence.

Similar to Cinnamon, Cassia dispels fear and replaces it with self-assurance. It challenges an individual to try even when they are afraid of making mistakes. Cassia aids those who feel foolish by helping them see their own brilliance. It supports the soul in seeing its own value and potential. Cassia assists the individual in discovering their innate gifts and talents. It invites the individual to "let their light shine" and live from their authentic self.

Suggested Uses: Place a few drops in a capsule and take internally. Dilute one drop with fractionated coconut oil and place over the solar plexus.

Emotions Addressed: Embarrassed, Hiding, Fear, Humiliated, Insecure, Judged, Shy, Worthless

Cinnamon

The Oil of Sexual Harmony

Cinnamon strongly supports the reproductive system and helps heal sexual issues. It assists individuals in accepting their body and embracing their physical attractiveness. Cinnamon dispels fear of rejection and nurtures healthy sexuality. It rekindles sexual energies when there has been repression, trauma or abuse. It can also bring clarity to souls who struggle with their sexual identity.

Cinnamon also assists individuals in relationships where insecurities are shown by jealousy and control. It encourages the soul to let go of control and allow others to be free. Cinnamon can nurture strong relationships based on mutual love and respect.

Where there are other insecurities covered by pretense, façade, and pride, Cinnamon invites individuals to be honest and vulnerable, thereby allowing true intimacy to emerge.

Suggested Uses: Place 3-5 drops in a capsule or glass of water. Inhale regularly.

Emotions Addressed: Body rejection, Fear, Controlling, Jealousy, Sexual Repression

Clary Sage

The Oil of Clarity & Vision

Clary Sage assists individuals in changing their perceptions. It gives courage to "see" the truth. One of the finest oils for the brow chakra, Clary Sage dispels darkness and illusion, helping a person to see their limiting belief systems. Clary Sage encourages individuals to remain open to new ideas and new perspectives. It can assist during a healing crisis when a drastic change of perspective is required. Clary Sage opens the soul to new possibilities and experiences.

Clary Sage assists in opening creative channels and clearing creative blocks. It eliminates distractions from the mind and assists individuals in finding a state of "emptiness" where creative forces may be realized. Opening us to the dream world, Clary Sage increases one's ability to visualize and imagine new possibilities.

Clary Sage teaches the spirit how to use its divinely given gifts and is especially helpful in clarifying spiritual vision. It assists in developing the gift of discernment. Clary Sage invites us to expand our vision and accept the reality of the spiritual world.

Suggested Uses: Place one drop on the forehead. Inhale regularly throughout the day.

Emotions Addressed: Confusion, "In the Dark," Discouragement, Disconnection from Spiritual Realms, Hopeless, Blocked Creativity

Clove

The Oil of Boundaries

Clove supports individuals in letting go of a "victim mentality." Victims feel overly influenced by other people and outside circumstances. They perceive themselves to be powerless to change their life situations. Clove supports individuals in standing up for themselves, being proactive and feeling capable of making their own choices, regardless of other's opinions or responses.

Clove assists the soul in letting go of patterns of self-betrayal and co-dependency by reconnecting an individual with their personal integrity. It builds up appropriate boundaries and defenses.

Clove gives the "pushover" the courage to say no. It reignites the inner soul fire and can assist anytime there has been damage to the Self related to childhood pain, trauma or abuse. Clove is especially helpful in breaking free of patterns of abuse by restoring the victim's sense of self and helping them regain the strength to stand up for their needs. Clove insists that we live true to ourselves and the Divine by establishing clear boundaries.

Suggested Uses: Place 3-5 drops oil in a capsule and take internally. Place 1-3 drops on feet and/or stomach.

Emotions Addressed: Victim, Defeated, Dominated, Enslaved, Fear of Rejection, Intimidated

Coriander

The Oil of Loyalty

Coriander is the oil of loyalty, specifically loyalty to self. The person in need of Coriander oil may be trapped in a cycle of serving others while neglecting their own needs. They may also have a strong need to do what is "right" or "correct." Often the mind's perspective of the "right" way is too limited and seen from only one perspective. Coriander reminds us that there is more than one way to do something and that fitting in often means we are not being true to the Self.

Coriander moves us from doing things for the acceptance of others to honoring and living from the true self. There are as many ways of "being" as there are people in the world. Each soul must learn its own way of living and being. Coriander gives courage to step out of the "box" and to risk being who we really are.

Coriander teaches us that we are each a gift to the world with something unique that no one else has to offer. Only we can be and express our uniqueness. Loyalty to the self means living in connection with what our spirit urges and directs. Coriander shifts individuals from needing others' acceptance to honoring and living from the true Self.

Suggested Uses: Place one drop on the forehead.

Emotions Addressed: Controlled by others, Self-betrayal, Drudgery, Conforming

Cypress

The Oil of Motion & Flow

This powerful oil creates energetic flow and emotional catharsis. Stagnant energies are brought into motion through the fluid energy of this oil. Cypress works in the heart and mind creating flexibility.

Cypress teaches us how to let go of the past by moving with the flow of life. This oil is especially indicated for individuals who are mentally or emotionally stuck, stiff, rigid, tense, over-striving or have perfectionistic tendencies. This "hard-driving" stems from fear and the need to control. The individual tries to force things in life rather than allowing them to unfold naturally.

Cypress encourages us to cast aside our worries and let go of control so we can enjoy the thrill that comes from being alive. It reminds us that "damnation" is simply the discontinuation of growth and development. Cypress shows us how to have perfect trust in the flow of life.

Suggested Uses: Inhale regularly throughout the day. Place 1-3 drops over the kidneys or just below the naval.

Emotions Addressed: Controlling, Fear, Perfectionism, Rigidity, Stuck, Tense

Eucalyptus

The Oil of Wellness

The strong medicinal aroma of Eucalyptus demonstrates it's powerful effect upon the physical and emotional bodies. Eucalyptus oil supports the soul who constantly faces illness. They may get well for times and seasons, only to return to a common cold, allergies or congestion in the sinuses and respiratory system.

Eucalyptus addresses a deep emotional/spiritual issue of "the need to be sick". It reveals patterns of thinking that continually create poor health. Such beliefs may include thoughts like "I don't deserve to be well," "I am the sort of person that is always getting sick," or "The only way I can get a break is to get sick." Eucalyptus gives an individual courage to face these issues and beliefs. It encourages them to let go of their attachments to illness.

Eucalyptus encourages individuals to take full responsibility for their own health. It bestows trust that individuals needs and desires can be met, even if they allow themselves to get well. Eucalyptus teaches the individual how to heal by claiming their wholeness.

Suggested Uses: Place 3-5 drops over chest, throat or spine and inhale regularly throughout the day.

Emotions Addressed: Attached to Illness, Clingy, Defeated, Despair, Want to Escape Life or Responsibilities, Imprisoned, Powerless to Heal, Sickly

Fennel

The Oil of Responsibility

Fennel supports the individual who has a weakened sense of "self". The individual may feel defeated by life's responsibilities, having little to no desire to improve their situation. Fennel reignites a passion for life. It encourages the soul to take full ownership and responsibility for its choices. Fennel teaches that life is not too much or too big to handle.

Fennel encourages an individual to live in integrity with themselves, despite the judgments of others. When one has been paralyzed by fear and shame, this oil gets them moving again. Fennel re-establishes a strong connection to the body and the "self" when there has been weakness or separation.

Fennel also supports an individual in listening to the subtle messages of the body. This is especially important in situations where there has been a loss of connection to the body's natural signals due to emotional eating, severe dieting, eating disorders or drug abuse. Through attunement with the body's actual needs, Fennel curbs cravings for experiences that dull the senses. This oil then supports the individual in *hearing* the body's signals of hunger, thirst, satiation, tiredness, or exhaustion. Fennel is also supportive in regaining one's appetite for nourishment, food and life itself.

Suggested Uses: Place a drop under the tongue after meals.

Emotions Addressed: Lack of Desire, Unwilling to Take Responsibility for Self/Life, Shame, Weak Sense of "Self"

Frankincense

The Oil of Truth

Frankincense reveals deceptions and false truths. It invites the individual to let go of lower vibrations, lies, deceptions and negativity. This oil helps create new perspectives based on light and truth. Frankincense recalls to memory spiritual understanding, gifts, wisdom and knowledge the soul brought into the world. It is a powerful cleanser of spiritual darkness. Frankincense assists in pulling the "scales of darkness" from the eyes, the barriers from the mind, and the walls from the heart. Through connecting the soul with its inner light, this oil reveals the truth.

Frankincense supports in creating a healthy attachment with one's father. It also assists in spiritual awakening. It helps an individual feel the fatherly love of the Divine. When one has felt abandoned or forgotten, Frankincense reminds them that they are loved and protected. While this oil is incredibly powerful, it is also gentle like a loving father who nurtures, guides and protects. Frankincense shields the body and soul from negative influences, and assists the soul in its spiritual evolution. Enhancing practices of prayer and meditation, this oil opens spiritual channels that allow an individual to connect spiritually. Through the light and power of Frankincense, the individual can draw closer to divinity, healthy masculinity and the grandeur of the True Self.

Suggested Uses: Place 1 drop under the tongue morning and night. Inhale regularly throughout the day.

Emotions Addressed: Abandonment, Spiritually Disconnected, Distant from Father, Unprotected

Geranium

The Oil of Love & Trust

Geranium restores confidence in the innate goodness of others and in the world. It facilitates trust, especially when an individual has lost trust in others due to difficult life circumstances. It also assists in re-establishing a strong bond to one's mother and father. When there has been a loss of trust in relationships, geranium encourages emotional honesty, love and forgiveness. It fosters receptivity to human love and connection.

Geranium heals the broken heart. It encourages emotional honesty by facilitating the emergence of grief or pain that has been suppressed. Geranium softens anger and assists in healing emotional wounds. It assists in re-opening the heart so that love may flow freely. Indeed, Geranium could be called "the emotional healer."

Geranium is a gentle oil, perfect for babies and children. It nurtures the inner-child and supports in re-parenting this aspect of the self. The individual who has a difficult time accessing their emotions can be supported by Geranium, as it leads individuals away from the logical mind and into the warmth and nurture of the heart. At its root, Geranium heals the heart, instills unconditional love, and fosters trust.

Suggested Uses: Place 1-3 drops on heart. Inhale regularly throughout the day.

Emotions Addressed: Addresses almost all types of emotional issues, including: Abandonment, Loss, Distrusting, Unforgiving, Unloving, Disheartened, Heavy Hearted, Grief

Ginger

The Oil of Empowerment

Ginger oil holds no reservations. It has a purpose, and it *will* fulfill it! Ginger powerfully persuades individuals to be fully present and participate in life. It teaches that to be successful in life we must be fully committed to it.

Ginger addresses deep patterns of victim mentality. A victim mentality is evidenced by feelings of powerlessness, believing everything is outside an individual's control, refusing to take responsibility for life, or blaming life circumstances on other people or outside influences. The victim feels "stuck," as they decentralize responsibility and blame others for their misfortunes.

Ginger empowers individuals in taking complete responsibility for their life circumstances. It infuses a warrior-like mentality based on personal integrity, centralized responsibility, and individual choice. Here, the individual sees themselves as the creator of their own life. No longer waiting on outside circumstances, they choose their own destiny. The empowered individual assumes full responsibility and accountability for the consequences of their actions or inactions.

Suggested Uses: Place 1-3 drops on stomach or take internally in a capsule. Inhale regularly throughout the day.

Emotions Addressed: Victim, Powerless, Unwilling to Take Responsibility for Self or Life, Defeated, Not Present

Grapefruit

The Oil of Honoring the Body

Grapefruit teaches true respect and appreciation for one's physical body. It supports individuals who struggle to honor their physical body and are caught in patterns of mistreatment. These forms of abuse may include severe dieting, judging one's body weight and type, and abusing the body through negligent behavior or violence. These acts are often motivated by a hate and disgust buried within the psyche which gets directed toward the physical body. Though the individual may obsess over how they look, deep down they never feel they look good enough. There is a dissatisfaction that persists.

Grapefruit oil is often misused in strict dietary and weight-loss programs. The reason this oil helps curb emotional eating is because it encourages a positive relationship with one's physical body based on love, tolerance and acceptance. Grapefruit encourages integrity by respecting one's physical needs. This oil assists an individual in listening to their true physical needs and impulses. It also assists one in taking responsibility for what they feel. Grapefruit teaches that no amount of food can fill a hole in the heart; only love can do that. As the individual takes ownership of their feelings and gets the help they need in addressing them, they no longer have a need to hide their feelings behind food, body abuse, strict regimens, eating disorders or other forms of addiction.

Suggested Uses: Place 1 drop under the tongue or in glass of water. Inhale regularly throughout the day.

Emotions Addressed: Hate for the Body, Addiction to Food or Dieting, Eating Disorders, Anxiety over Appearance

Helichrysum

The Oil for Pain

Helichrysum removes pain quickly and effortlessly. It aids "the walking wounded" – those with a history of difficult life circumstances, trauma, addiction, loss or abuse. These ... pport that ... endurance to the ... despite past ... n life and in the self, ..." Helichrysum has ... he sun. It imbues ... sum takes the ... through life's ... n persevere, this oil ... al consciousness.

... formation, ... ave gratitude for ... y were not wounded, ... eby experiencing spiritual rebirth. Just as the phoenix dies and is raised from its ashes, so might an individual be raised from their turmoil. Helichrysum lends its warrior spirit so that one may face their adversities with courage and determination. It brings hope to the most discouraged of souls and life to those in need of rebirth.

Suggested Uses: Place 1-3 drops over the heart and/or along spine. Inhale regularly throughout the day.

Emotions Addressed: Intense Pain, Anguish, Turmoil

Handwritten notes:
Sleep
- 1 drop on each footarch
- 1 drop on forehead & rub clockwise
- 1 drop behind neck

Lavender

The Oil of Communication

Lavender aids verbal expression. It calms the insecurities that are felt when one risks their true thoughts and feelings. Lavender addresses a deep fear of being seen and heard. Individuals in need of Lavender hide within, blocking all forms of true self-expression. While they may even be going through the motions of outward expression, they're actually holding back because the expression is not connected to the heart or soul.

Lavender supports individuals in releasing the tension and constriction that stems from fear of expressing one's self. Due to past experiences, they may believe it is not safe to express themselves. The true Self is therefore trapped within and goes unexpressed. Strong feelings of being unlovable, unimportant, or unheard accompany this condition. The individual's fear of rejection paralyzes their true voice and traps their feelings inside.

Lavender encourages emotional honesty and insists that we speak our innermost thoughts and desires. As individuals learn to communicate their deepest thoughts and feelings, they are liberated from their self-inflicted prison. It is through open and honest communication that an individual experiences unconditional love and acceptance. Through Lavender's courageous spirit, we are free to share our true self with others.

Suggested Uses: Place 1-3 drops on throat. Inhale regularly throughout the day.

Emotions Addressed: Blocked communication, Fear of Rejection, Feeling Unseen or Unheard, Constricted

Lemon

The Oil of Focus

The delightful citrusy aroma of Lemon oil nourishes the mind and aids concentration. While Lemon supports the emotional body, its major effects are experienced in the mental field. The crisp scent of Lemon oil improves one's ability to focus. Lemon is a wonderful aid for children struggling with school. It teaches individuals to be mentally present by focusing on one thing at a time. Lemon dispels confusion and bestows clarity. It counterbalances mental fatigue due to too much study or reading. Lemon restores energy, mental flexibility, and drive to complete a project.

Lemon is especially helpful in cases of learning disorders. Whether an individual has a difficult time concentrating or feels incapable of learning, Lemon clears self-judgments about learning such as "I'm dumb" or "I am not a good student." Lemon calms fears and insecurities while restoring confidence in the self.

Emotionally, Lemon inspires a natural playfulness and buoyancy in the heart. It assists in releasing feelings of depression by restoring feelings of joy and happiness. Lemon inspires joyful involvement in the present moment by infusing energy, confidence and alertness in the soul.

Suggested Uses: Place 1-3 drops on stomach and behind ears. Place 1 drop in glass of water. Inhale regularly throughout the day.

Emotions Addressed: Confusion, Inability to Focus, Mental fatigue, Lack of Joy and Energy, Learning Disorders, Guilt

Lemongrass

The Oil of Cleansing

Lemongrass is a powerful cleanser of energy. It dispels feelings of despondency, despair and lethargy. Lemongrass assists individuals in entering a healing mode or cleansing state. In this state, one easily lets go of old, limiting beliefs, toxic energies and negativity. Lemongrass teaches individuals to move forward without hesitation. It asks them to commit to a healing path where change is a regular occurrence.

Lemongrass can also be a powerful tool in cleansing the energy within a house, room or office space. It can give the individual with "pack rat" tendencies courage to let go of old things. Lemongrass asks authoritatively that we let go of everything we no longer need.

Lemongrass also supports the brow chakra or "spiritual eyes" in cleansing negative energy. As an individual lets go of past issues and old baggage, they have an increased ability to see things with greater clarity. Lemongrass supports an individual's energy in flowing freely and smoothly. Lemongrass has a powerful mission in assisting individuals to cleanse physically, emotionally and spiritually.

Suggested Uses: Place 1-3 drops over kidneys. Inhale regularly throughout the day. Place 10 drops in a spray bottle and mist around house or room.

Emotions Addressed: Toxic or Negative Energy, Darkness, Despair, Holding on to the Past, Hoarding, Spiritual Blindness

Lime

The Oil of Zest for Life

Lime imbues the soul with a zest for life. When an individual has been weighed down by discouragement or grief, Lime elevates them above the mire. It instills courage and cheer in the heart, and reminds one to be grateful for the gift of life.

Lime cleanses the heart, especially when there has been an accumulation of emotional toxins due to avoidance or repression. This oil revitalizes the heart space, giving room for light and joy. It clears discouragement, depression and suicidal thoughts and feelings. Lime shines light on the inner motives hidden in the heart, and encourages emotional honesty.

Lime can also assist the individual who has overly developed their intellectual capacities but has neglected to develop themselves emotionally. This oil encourages balance between the heart and mind. It clears congestion powerfully from the heart region so that one may feel safe with their feelings and at home in their heart. Lime dispels apathy and resignation and instills hope, joy, courage, and the determination to face all of life's challenges.

Suggested Uses: Place 1-3 drops on chest. Inhale regularly throughout the day.

Emotions Addressed: Apathy, Resignation, Grief, Suicidal Thoughts and Feelings, Discouragement

Marjoram

The Oil of Connection

Marjoram aids those who are unable to trust others or form meaningful relationships. This inability to trust often stems from harsh life experiences. The individual develops a fear of close connection in human relationships. They may tend towards reclusive behaviors, protecting themselves even further by abstaining from social interactions. They may also protect themselves by unconsciously sabotaging long-term relationships. Marjoram shows the barriers they have formed to protect themselves from others. It reveals patterns of aloofness, distancing one's self from other people, or being "cold." Those in need of Marjoram oil most likely use these protective coping strategies unintentionally. Deep down they desire the intimate connection they subconsciously sabotage.

Marjoram teaches that trust is the basis for all human relationships. It assists an individual in increasing their warmth and trust in social situations. Marjoram softens the heart and heals past wounds. It kindles the fires of trust in relationships so that one may "blossom." When an individual feels safe and loved, they express their authenticity. Marjoram restores trust and openness so that true bonds of love may be formed in friendships and relationships.

Suggested Uses: Place 1-3 drops over the heart. Inhale regularly throughout the day.

Emotions Addressed: Distrust, Aloof, Protected, Distant, Emotional Isolation, Reclusive, "Cold"

Melaleuca

The Oil of Energetic Boundaries

Disinfectant by nature, Melaleuca, also known as "tea tree oil," clears negative energetic baggage. It specifically releases co-dependent and parasitic relationships. These toxic relationships may be with people, microorganisms in the physical body, or spiritual beings. The individual may feel drained of life-force and energy, but they may not be consciously aware of the source of this energy leakage. Melaleuca helps break the negative ties in these kinds of relationships so that new, healthy connections may be formed with people who honor one's personal space and boundaries. This energetic "vampirism" between organisms violates the laws of nature. Melaleuca encourages an individual to only connect to people and beings that honor and respect others' agency. It helps the individual to recognize the parts of themselves that nurtured, allowed, and perhaps even encouraged such relationships to exist in the first place.

Through these empowering processes, Melaleuca encourages an individual to relinquish all forms of self-betrayal, including: allowing others to take advantage of one's time, energy, or talents, "doormat" tendencies, letting others "feed" on one's energy, not standing up for the self, being weak-willed or feeling responsible for the problems of others. It assists an individual in purification practices and in releasing toxic debris.

Suggested Uses: Place a drop under the tongue. Inhale regularly throughout the day.

Emotions Addressed: Parasitic and Co-dependent Relationships, Poor Boundaries, Weak Willed, Toxicity

Melissa

The Oil of Light

Melissa oil awakens the soul to truth and light. It reminds them of who they truly are and why they came to this earth. Melissa invites one to release everything and anything that holds them back from reaching their fullest potential.

Melissa assists an individual in receiving spiritual guidance by re-connecting them with their inner voice. It uplifts the soul on all levels by literally preparing one to "up-level." When an individual feels too weighed-down by the burdens of life, Melissa encourages them to keep going. It gives strength and vitality to the innermost recesses of the heart and soul. This oil invites one to participate in higher realms of living and dreaming. As an individual stays connected to spiritual sources, they feel a lightness in their being and a brightness in their core. Melissa reminds one that every individual has a "spark" of divinity within them, and that with love and attention, that spark will grow. This oil fuels that spark of energy, igniting an individual's True Self. Melissa assists them in shedding everything that is not in harmony with that inner-light.

Melissa's enthusiasm is contagious. Through the intense light and vibration Melissa has to offer, an individual may feel they cannot help but let go of depression and other low vibrations that are holding them down. It teaches one of the joy of living.

Suggested Uses: Place 1 drop on the thumb and place on the roof of mouth. Inhale regularly throughout the day.

Emotions Addressed: Depression, Darkened, Dreary, Suicidal

Myrrh

The Oil of Mother Earth

Myrrh oil nurtures the soul's relationship with the maternal mother and with the earth. This oil supports individuals who have had disturbances with the mother-child bond. Whether it is a division between the child and the biological mother or whether it be mother earth herself, Myrrh can help bridge the gap and heal the disturbance. This division, or lack of attachment may be related to adoption, birth trauma, malnourishment, experiences of abandonment, or other childhood issues. Myrrh helps the soul to feel the love and nurturing presence of "Mother." Similar to nutrient-rich colostrum found in a mother's milk, Myrrh oil inoculates individuals from the adverse and harmful effects of the world. Like the warmth of a mother's love for her child, Myrrh assists individuals in feeling safe and secure.

When the mother-child bond has been disrupted, the soul may lose it childlike ability to trust. Feelings of trust are replaced with feelings of fear and a belief that the world is unsafe. Myrrh assists individuals in letting go of fear. Through reestablishing a healthy connection to the earth and to one's own mother, Myrrh rekindles trust within the soul. As the individual learns to once again live in trust, confidence in the goodness of life returns and the soul feels more safe and at home on the earth.

Suggested Uses: Place 1-3 drops on bottom of feet and heart. Inhale regularly throughout the day.

Emotions Addressed: Distrust of Others, Feeling Unsafe in the World, Disrupted Maternal Connection, Malnourished

Orange, Wild

The Oil of Abundance

Wild Orange addresses a wider variety of emotional issues than any other essential oil. It inspires abundance, fosters creativity, supports a positive mood, restores physical energy, and aids in transitions. Wild Orange also reconnects individuals with their inner child and brings spontaneity, fun, joy and play into one's life.

At its core, Wild Orange teaches the true meaning of abundance. It encourages individuals to let go of a scarcity mindset with all of its manifestations, including: fear, nervousness, inflexibility, workaholism, lack of humor, and the belief that there is not enough. Wild Orange reminds the soul of the limitless supply found in nature. Fruit trees, like wild orange, give freely to all in need. Wild Orange teaches us to give without thought of compensation. In nature, there is always enough to go around. Wild Orange encourages individuals to let go of their need to hoard, which is the epitome of scarcity.

Wild Orange also assists an individual's natural creative sense. It inspires limitless solutions for problems and issues. We never need to fear. Wild Orange invites us to completely let go as a child does and to live from our authentic self. In our authenticity, we *are* abundance. Sharing, playing, relaxing, and enjoying the bounties of life; these are the gifts bestowed by Wild Orange.

Suggested Uses: Place 1-3 drops on stomach or just below the naval. Inhale regularly throughout the day.

Emotions Addressed: Scarcity, Over-Seriousness, Rigid, Dull, Workaholism, Low Energy, Discouraged

Oregano

The Oil of Humility & Non-Attachment

Oregano cuts through the "fluff" of life and teaches us to do the same. It removes blocks, clears negativity, and cuts away negative attachments. Oregano is a powerful oil and may even be called "forceful" or "intense."

Oregano addresses a person's need to be "right." The individual in need of Oregano may attempt to convert other people to their own fixed opinions. Their strong will often makes them unteachable and unwilling to budge. They hold rigidly to their opinions and belief systems. However, Oregano is resolute, as it takes a powerful oil to break through a strong will.

On the deepest level, Oregano dispels materialism and attachment that hinders an individual's growth and progress. While using Oregano, a person may feel encouraged to end a toxic relationship, quit an oppressive job, or end a lifelong addiction. These toxic attachments limit one's capacities to feel a healthy connection to the Divine. Oregano encourages true spirituality by inviting us to live in non-attachment. It teaches that devotion to our Higher Power includes letting go of rigidity, willfulness, negative attachments and materialism.

Suggested Uses: Place 5-7 drops in a capsule and take internally. Inhale regularly throughout the day.

Emotions Addressed: Overly Attached, Pride, Opinionated, Negative, Excessively Willful

Patchouli

The Oil of Physicality

Patchouli supports individuals in becoming fully present in the physical body. It balances those who feel devitalized and who seek to escape the body through spiritual pursuits or other forms of distraction. Patchouli tempers the obsessive personality by bringing them "down" to reality and teaching them moderation. It is grounding and stabilizing.

Patchouli compliments yoga practice, tai chi, or other exercises that aim to connect the spirit and the body. While using Patchouli, individuals feel more grounded and fluid. This oil calms fears and nervous tension, stilling the heart and mind in preparing the spirit and body for deeper union. It also helps individuals to stay in touch with the earth.

Patchouli helps individuals to appreciate the magnificence of the physical body and all of its natural processes and functions. It assists in releasing emotional judgments and issues related to the body, such as believing the body is unholy or dirty. This oil helps with body image distortions and general body dislike. Patchouli brings confidence in the body, as well as grace, poise and physical strength. It reminds the individual of childhood experiences of using the body for play and fun. On the deepest level, Patchouli assists an individual to feel at peace while being present in their physical body.

Suggested Uses: Place 1-3 drops on bottom of feet and just below the navel. Inhale regularly throughout the day.

Emotions Addressed: Body Shame, Disconnect from the Body, Judgment of the Body, Tension in Body

Peppermint

The Oil of a Buoyant Heart

Peppermint brings joy and buoyancy to the heart and soul. It invigorates body, mind and spirit. It reminds us that life can be happy, and there is nothing to fear. It lifts an individual out of their emotional trials for a short reprieve. When an individual uses Peppermint, they feel as though they're gliding through life. It assists in staying on the surface of emotional issues like a water skier on a lake. The power of Peppermint can be felt most in times of discouragement or depression. When the individual is disheartened, they may use Peppermint to re-discover the joy of being alive.

However, a person may also abuse the properties of Peppermint oil. If Peppermint is used as a permanent escape to avoid dealing with emotional pain, it can hinder growth and progress. Peppermint should not be used in this way. It aids individuals who need a short "breather." At times, a reprieve is necessary before re-entering emotional waters, but we are not meant to wade in the shallow end forever. When it is accepted and embraced, emotional pain serves as our teacher. Peppermint can assist an individual in regaining the strength needed to face their emotional reality.

Suggested Uses: Place 1-3 drops over the heart or on stomach. Inhale regularly throughout the day.

Emotions Addressed: Unbearable Pain, Intense Depression, Heaviness, Pessimistic, Muddled

Roman Chamomile

The Oil of Spiritual Purpose

Roman Chamomile supports individuals in discovering and living their true life purpose. Regardless of what we do for a living, Chamomile can help us to find purpose and meaning in our lives. As we live from the center of our being, we find a power and a purpose that is indescribable. We feel more at peace and more calm. Chamomile softens the personality, easing the overactive ego-mind. It restores our confidence to do what we came here to do. Like a guardian angel, Chamomile leads us to where we need to be and what we need to be doing.

Roman Chamomile assists a person in shedding the meaningless activities that consume their lives so that they can focus on a more fulfilling work, even the work of their own souls. Chamomile assists us in feeling connected to and supported by divine helpers and guides. It calms our insecurities about following our spiritual path. People fear and believe that if they do what they love, they will end up destitute. Roman Chamomile says, "Do what you love and everything will be a success."

Suggested Uses: Place 1-3 drops over the stomach, on the brow or behind ears. Inhale regularly throughout the day.

Emotions Addressed: Purposeless, Discouraged, Drudgery, Frustration, Unsettled

Rose

The Oil of Divine Love

Rose oil holds a higher frequency than any other oil on the planet. It is a powerful healer of the heart. It supports an individual in reaching heavenward and contacting Divine love. Rose teaches the essential need for Divine grace and intervention in the healing process. As an individual opens to receive Divine benevolence in all its manifestations, the heart is softened. If one can simply "let go" and choose to receive Divine love, they are wrapped in warmth, charity and compassion.

Rose invites individuals to experience the unwavering, unchanging, unconditional love of the Divine. This love heals all hearts and dresses all wounds. It restores an individual to authenticity, wholeness and purity. As one feels unconditional love and acceptance, the heart is softened. As the heart is fully opened, a fountain of love flows freely through the soul. In this state, one feels charity and compassion. Charity is experienced on behalf of one's self and others. Rose embodies Divine love, and teaches individuals how to contact this love through prayer, meditation, and opening the heart to receive.

Suggested Uses: Place one drop over the heart or inhale as needed.

Emotions Addressed: Bereft of Divine Love, Constricted Feelings, Closed or Broken Heart, Lack of Brotherly Love

Rosemary

The Oil of Knowledge & Transition

Rosemary assists in the development of true knowledge and true intellect. It teaches that we can be instructed from a far greater space of understanding than the human mind. It challenges us to look deeper than we normally would, and ask more soul-searching questions so that we may receive more inspired answers.

Rosemary also assists individuals who struggle with learning disabilities. It brings expansion to the mind, supporting individuals in receiving new information and new experiences.

Rosemary aids in times of transition and change. When a person is having a difficult time adjusting to a new house, school, or relationship, Rosemary can assist. It teaches that we do not understand all things because we have a mortal perspective. Rosemary invites us to trust in a higher, more intelligent power than ourselves. It supports us in feeling confident and assured during times of great change in understanding or perspective. Rosemary roots us in the true knowledge that surpasses all understanding.

Suggested Uses: Place 1-3 drops on the brow, the neck or behind the ears. Inhale regularly throughout the day.

Emotions Addressed: Confusion, Difficulty Adjusting/Transitioning, Ignorance

Sandalwood

The Oil of Sacred Devotion

Sandalwood assists with all kinds of prayer, meditation and spiritual worship. It teaches reverence and respect for Deity. This oil has been used since ancient times for its powerful ability to calm the mind, still the heart, and prepare the spirit to commune with God.

Sandalwood teaches of spiritual devotion and spiritual sacrifice. It invites us to place all material attachments on the altar of sacrifice so that we may truly progress spiritually. This oil asks us where our hearts are and challenges us to re-order our priorities to be in alignment with the Divine will.

Sandalwood assists us in quieting our minds so that we may hear the subtle voice of the Spirit. It raises individuals into higher levels of consciousness. Sandalwood assists us in reaching beyond our current confines and belief systems. For those who are ready to leave behind fame, wealth and the need for acceptance, Sandalwood teaches true humility, devotion, and love for the Divine.

Suggested Uses: Place a drop over the brow area. Inhale before meditation, study or prayer.

Emotions Addressed: Disconnected from God or Spiritual Self, Emptiness, Over-thinking, Materialism

Thyme

The Oil of Releasing & Forgiving

Thyme is one of the most powerful cleansers of the emotional body, and assists in addressing trapped feelings which have been buried for a long time. It reaches deep within the body and soul, searching for unresolved negativity. Thyme brings to the surface old, stagnant feelings. It is particularly helpful in treating the toxic emotions of hate, rage, anger and resentment, which cause the heart to close.

Thyme empties the soul of all negativity, leaving the heart wide open. In this state of openness, an individual begins to feel tolerance and patience for others. As the heart opens more and more, it is able to receive love and offer forgiveness. Thyme teaches, "It's time to move forward and let go." As an individual forgives, they free themselves from emotional bondage. Thyme transforms hate and anger into love and forgiveness.

Suggested Uses: Place 5-6 drops in a capsule and take internally. Inhale regularly throughout the day.

Emotions Addressed: Unforgiving Heart, Anger, Rage, Hate, Bitterness, Resentment

Vetiver

The Oil of Centering & Descent

Vetiver oil assists us in becoming more "rooted" in life. Life can scatter one's energy and cause one to feel split between different priorities, people and activities. Vetiver brings the individuals back down to earth. It assists them in "grounding" to the physical world. Vetiver also assists individuals in deeply connecting with what they think and feel. In this way, the oil is incredibly supportive in all kinds of self-awareness work. It encourages uncovering the root of an emotional issue.

Vetiver challenges individuals' need to escape their pain. It centers them in Self and guides them downward to the root of their emotional issues. It helps them find relief, but not through avoidance. Relief comes after they have traveled within and met the core of their emotional issue. Vetiver will not let them quit. It grounds them in the present moment and carries them through an emotional catharsis. The descent into the Self assists individuals in discovering deeper facets of their being. Vetiver opens the doors to light and recovery through this "downward journey."

Suggested Uses: Place 1-3 drops on feet. Inhale regularly throughout the day.

Emotions Addressed: Apathetic, Despondent, Disconnected, Scattered, Split, Stressed

Prof. Dr. S. Freud
Wien IX, Berggasse 19.
Telephon 14362.   Sprechst. 3—5.

White Fir
Purify
Roman Chamomile
Vetiver

© E

50

White Fir

The Oil of Generational Healing

White Fir addresses "generational" issues. Patterns and traditions are passed down from family member to family member. Some of these patterns are positive, while others are negative and destructive. Examples of these negative patterns include: addiction, abuse, alcoholism, anger, co-dependency, eating disorders, pride, the need to be right, etc.

White Fir assists the individual in unearthing these negative patterns from the hidden recesses of the body and soul. As they are brought to the light of consciousness, they can be put to rest. The individual can choose not to participate in destructive family patterns and thereby break the tradition. White Fir aids this process and increases an individual's chances of success. In breaking these patterns, it offers a refuge of spiritual protection and helps individuals stay true to the path of healing, even if their family members oppose them in leaving behind their traditions.

Suggested Uses: Place 1-3 drops over chest or feet. Inhale regularly throughout the day.

Emotions Addressed: Feelings that are "Generational" or "Hereditary," Burdened by the Issues of Others

Wintergreen

The Oil of Surrender

Wintergreen is the oil of surrender. It can assist the strong-willed individual in letting go of the need to "know" and the need to be "right." It takes great strength to surrender to one's Higher Power. Wintergreen imbues the soul with this strength and teaches how to "let go" and be free of the negativity and pain which the soul holds on to. The need to be "right" in believing that life is painful will make it so. The need to be "right" in believing that we have to do life on our own will make that true as well.

Yet, Wintergreen reminds us that we do not have to do life on our own. There is always an invitation to surrender our burdens to our Higher Power. All that is required of us is to release and let go. Wintergreen teaches us that we can turn our hardships over to that Power greater than ourselves so that we do not have to carry the burden of life all alone.

Suggested Uses: Place 1-3 drops over the kidneys. Inhale regularly throughout the day.

Emotions Addressed: Need to Control, Feeling Weak, Willful

Ylang Ylang

The Oil of the Inner Child

Ylang Ylang is a powerful remedy for the heart. Modern-day society honors and reveres the mind over the heart and its intuitive ways of receiving information. Ylang Ylang brings the individual back to childhood and to the simple ways of the heart. This oil is about play and restoring a childlike nature and innocence to one's life. It assists in reaching deeply into "heart knowing."

Ylang Ylang is also a powerful remedy for releasing emotional trauma from the past. It is therefore a fantastic support in age regression work and other methods of healing. Ylang Ylang can assist one in releasing bottled-up emotions such as anger and sadness. Feelings that have been buried inside are easily brought to the light through Ylang Ylang's assistance. This oil allows emotional healing to flow naturally, nurturing the heart through the process. It reminds the individual that joy can be felt and experienced more fully by allowing them to feel a full range of emotions.

Suggested Uses: Place 1-3 drops over the heart. Inhale regularly throughout the day.

Emotions Addressed: Joylessness, Over-stressed, Grief, Sadness, Loss of a Loved One

OIL BLENDS

AromaTouch Blend

The Oil of Relaxation

dōTERRA's AromaTouch blend was formulated for massage. This specific combination of oils assists the body in calming, relaxing and releasing physical tension. On an emotional level, AromaTouch moves an individual from stiffness of heart and mind to openness and flexibility. AromaTouch is soothing to both the body and the mind. It comforts in times of grief and sorrow.

Most people seek out massage when they are tense or stressed. Through bodywork and massage the individual is able to relax their tight muscles. Breathing may begin to regulate, slow and deepen. As an individual's body relaxes, so does their mind. As the muscles release tension, the heart can reopen to life. Circulation is enhanced, as is their ability to move with life and allow things to flow. This is the gift of AromaTouch; the ability to relax, open and move in harmony once more with the body and with existence.

Ingredients: Basil, Grapefruit, Cypress, Marjoram, Lavender, Peppermint,

Suggested Uses: Place 1-3 drop over the spine or tight muscles. Inhale regularly throughout the day.

Emotions Addressed: Tense, Stiffness in Body or Mind, Stressed

Balance Blend

The Oil of Grounding

dōTERRA's Balance blend was formulated for grounding the body. Balance oil is primarily a combination of tree oils. Trees live in the present moment. They are not in a hurry. They are stable. Balance oil's soft energy is excellent for calming hyperactive children who have difficulty settling down. It is also a wonderful remedy for adults who need to reconnect with their roots. Balance oil strengthens a connection with the lower body and with the earth. This connection is especially important when the upper faculties have been overused due to excessive thinking, speaking, or spiritual activity.

Balance oil is especially suited for personalities who seek to escape from life through disconnection or disassociation. These individuals may avoid long-term commitments in work or relationships, preferring instead to "drift" with the wind. Balance reminds individuals that to realize their true dreams and desires, an individual must stay focused on a goal until it is actualized in the physical world. Balance teaches true perseverance by staying present with a specific plan or idea until it is embodied. Balance provides inner strength and fortitude. It teaches an individual to ground their energy and to manifest their vision with the patience of a tree.

Ingredients: Spruce, Rosewood, Blue Tansy, Frankincense

Suggested Uses: Place 3-6 drops on bottoms of the feet. Inhale regularly throughout the day.

Emotions Addressed: Lack of Desire, Unwilling to take Responsibility for self/life, Shame, Weak Sense of "Self"

Breathe Blend

The Oil of Breath

dōTERRA's Breathe blend was formulated for the respiratory system. The person in need of Breathe oil wants everything to proceed rapidly. Feeling rushed, they hasten their breathing to match their mental pace. As the mind is deprived of oxygen, foggy headedness ensues. The over-active mind, coupled with shallow breathing, creates a high-strung state. The individual may have a hard time relaxing due to the patterns of over-stimulation. They struggle to let go of obsessive thoughts and worries and don't feel they have time to "take a deep breath." We can intentionally trigger relaxation by slowing down our breathing. Breathe addresses a state of burnout and fatigue due to excessive thinking and weakened breathing.

The oils in Breathe have powerful effects on the lungs and air passages. Breath supports our connection to our spirit, and our connection to all life. Many forms of stress and depression are caused by shallow breathing. Emotionally, Breathe essential oil relates to our ability to take in life. It invites us to continually let go (breathe out) and then receive (breathe in). Breathe essential oil, in combination with more oxygen revitalizes our whole system. It imbues us with vigor, energy and enthusiasm.

Ingredients: Laurel Leaf (Bay), Peppermint, Eucalyptus radiata, Melaleuca alternifolia, Lemon, Ravensara

Suggested Uses: Place 1-3 drops on chest. Inhale regularly throughout the day.

Emotions Addressed: Hurried, Cannot Take a Deep Breath, Anxious

Citrus Bliss Blend

The Oil of Creativity

dōTERRA's Citrus Bliss blend is helpful for individuals who are overly-emotional to the point of imbalance. Citrus Bliss acts as a powerful "fire starter." It returns motivation and drive when it is lacking. This is a wonderful oil for addressing lethargy, discouragement, despondency, or low will to live. When the soul has lost its connection to the magic in life, Citrus Bliss helps restore the spark.

Citrus Bliss inspires creativity. Every human soul has a need to create. Citrus Bliss inspires this creative expression. It re-connects individuals with their inner-child and their natural creative sense. It inspires individuals to live abundantly and spontaneously. This combination of citrus oils encourages play and excitement. Citrus Bliss inspires us to use our true creative power by letting go of old limitations and insecurities. It takes courage to put one's self out there artistically. Citrus Bliss brings color and imagination to one's life. It invites us to quit smothering our creative energies and allow them to flow freely. Placed over the solar plexus, Citrus Bliss restores confidence in one's self and in one's creations. Citrus bliss rekindles the fire of the personality and fills the heart with creativity and with joy.

Ingredients: Wild Orange, Lemon, Grapefruit, Mandarin, Bergamot, Tangerine, Clementine, Vanilla Bean Extract

Suggested Uses: Place 1-3 drops over the solar plexus or on heart. Inhale regularly throughout the day.

Emotions Addressed: Stifled or Blocked Creativity, Fear of Self Expression, Emotionally Imbalanced, Low Will to Live

Clear Skin Blend

The Oil for Accepting Affliction

dōTERRA's Clear Skin blend was formulated for acne and general skin health. Its primary ingredient is black cumin seed oil, which is not an essential oil, but has small amounts of essential oil within in it. Black cumin is prized in many Islamic countries for its healing properties. The Prophet Muhammad said, "In black cumin seed there is a cure for every disease, except death."

Clear Skin emotionally supports individuals who struggle with skin related issues. These skin issues are often caused by suppressed anger, guilt or self-judgment. The individual in need of Clear Skin may sometimes feel like a victim or a martyr who may become overly absorbed in their pain and anguish. This pain and agony can quickly turn to blame and anger. The individual may lash out at other people or treat others with disdain, projecting their feelings of pain and inadequacy onto them.

Negative thinking literally "boils" to the surface of the skin as well as the external life. Clear Skin reverses the whole process by increasing self-love. It opens individuals to see their inherent worth. Clear Skin helps them look past menial imperfections and replace judgments with acceptance of one's self despite physical afflictions.

Ingredients: Black Cumin Seed Oil, Rosewood, Melaleuca, Eucalyptus, Geranium, Lemongrass

Suggested Uses: Rub on skin. Inhale regularly throughout the day.

Emotions Addressed: Absorbed in Afflictions

Deep Blue Blend

The Oil of Surrendering Pain

dōTERRA's Deep Blue assists individuals who are intensely resisting or avoiding their emotional pain. It gives a person strength to face their emotional wounds, allowing them to surface for transformation and healing. It teaches individuals how to be "the observer" of their painful experiences rather than becoming over-identified with them. When a person suffers from great emotional or physical pain, it is common for them to act irrationally or "lose their head." Deep Blue supports the mind in staying cool and collected, regardless of the emotional turmoil or physical pain one may be in. In this way, the individual maintains mental clarity in the face of danger and pain.

At the core level, Deep Blue teaches individuals acceptance and tolerance of their pain. It reveals the possibility that pain is not cruel, but is simply our teacher. Instead of resisting pain as a "bad" thing and something to be avoided, one may embrace the lessons it has to offer. As we let go of resistance, the pain lessens and often dissipates altogether. Pain, however, will not be ignored. Deep Blue invites us to accept pain as our teacher, release it, and let go of it.

Ingredients: Wintergreen, Camphor, Peppermint, Blue Tansy, Blue Chamomile, Helichrysum, Osmanthus

Suggested Uses: Place 1-3 drops on most painful physical location. Inhale regularly throughout the day.

Emotions Addressed: Resistance to Pain, Avoidance of Emotional Issues, Hysteria in Painful Situations

DigestZen

The Oil of Digestion

dōTERRA's DigestZen blend was formulated to support the body's digestive system. It also has a powerful emotional quality for supporting individuals who lack interest in life and the physical world. The individual may have a tendency to "bite off more than they can chew" by trying to do too much at once. This overload of information and stimulation may lead to an emotional form of "indigestion," where the individual cannot break down life experiences into palatable forms. The soul literally becomes overfed and undernourished, as it cannot translate their experiences into a usable form. When the individual is fully overwhelmed and over stimulated, they may lose their appetite for food, life and the physical world in general. They may become apathetic about their situation and begin neglecting their body's basic needs.

DigestZen combines the powerful oils of Ginger, Peppermint and other spices to support the body and the spirit in assimilating new information and events. It increases an individual's ability to receive new information, new relationships, and new experiences and be open to new possibilities. DigestZen powerfully aids individuals in digesting life's many experiences.

Ingredients: Ginger, Peppermint, Tarragon, Fennel, Caraway, Coriander, Anise

Suggested Uses: Place a drop under the tongue before or after meals. Inhale regularly throughout the day.

Emotions Addressed: Loss of Appetite in Food or Life, Inability to Assimilate New Information or Experiences

Elevation Blend

The Oil of Joy

dōTERRA's Elevation blend was formulated as an anti-depressant. This blend combines powerful mood stabilizers such as Sandalwood and Ylang Ylang with joy filled oils such as Tangerine, Elemi and Lemon Myrtle. The warm vibration of Melissa and Osmanthus oils in Elevation soothes the heart and balances the emotions.

Elevation can assist individuals in letting go of lower energy vibrations. Old habits and addictions lose their appeal as an individual shifts into higher levels of consciousness. Elevation raises our energy levels and energetic vibrations into higher states. It inspires feelings of: cheerfulness, brightness, courage, relaxation, happiness, humor, play and fun. By inspiring these feelings, Elevation transforms depression into sunshine and joy. It teaches us that worry and fear are not productive, but faith and hope and determination are. This oil powerfully persuades people to be happy, carefree and abundant. It supports us in flowing with life while remaining in peace and light.

Ingredients: Lavandin, Tangerine, Elemi, Lemon Myrtle, Melissa, Ylang Ylang, Osmanthus, Sandalwood

Suggested Uses: Place 1-3 drops over the brow. Inhale regularly throughout the day.

Emotions Addressed: Caught in Low Vibrations, Depression, Dark, Serious, Stern

Immortelle Blend

The Oil of Spiritual Insight

dōTERRA's Immortelle blend was formulated for skin health and longevity. However, this powerful combination of oils offers so much more. This blend combines the highest vibrational and most potent oils on the planet all into one blend. Although gentle, Immortelle powerfully assists individuals in shifting out of negativity, darkness and spiritual blindness.

Immortelle's powerful qualities may be felt most during the "dark night of the soul" when the individual experiences loss of identity, extreme paradigm shifts, and spiritual awakening all at once. Immortelle offers grace and comfort to the individual at this time, as well as anytime that one feels a loss of light, discouragement or distress. It offers true perspective on one's problems and issues by offering profound insight. During dark times, Immortelle assists individuals in feeling the grace and benevolence of the Divine. This powerful oil teaches that our intense anguish and emotional pain can catapult us into new heights of spiritual growth and development. Immortelle assists us in transcending the darkness in our lives. At its core, Immortelle raises levels of human consciousness and prepares individuals for new heights of spiritual transformation.

Ingredients: Frankincense, Sandalwood, Lavender, Myrrh, Helichrysum, Rose

Suggested Uses: Rub one drop on forehead. Inhale regularly throughout the day.

Emotions Addressed: Dark Night of the Soul, Spiritual Blindness, in the Dark, Lack of Insight

OnGuard Blend

The Oil of Protection

dōTERRA's OnGuard blend was formulated as a remedy to protect individuals from bacteria, mold and viruses. This blend's protective properties, however, extend beyond the physical level by aiding individuals in warding off energetic parasites, domineering personalities, and other negative influences. OnGuard strengthens one's immune system, which governs the ability to defend against attacks from physical pathogens or negative energies.

This blend is incredibly helpful for strengthening the inner-self along with the inner resolve to stand up for one's self and live in integrity. OnGuard is especially indicated for personalities who have a weakened boundary due to perpetual violation of some kind to their personal space. OnGuard gives the individual strength to say "no" and resolve to maintain clear boundaries. The individual literally feels stronger and more equipped to handle life's challenges. This blend cuts away unhealthy connections such as codependency, parasitic relationships or emotional viruses found in negative "group thought." OnGuard's physical and energetic protective qualities greatly assist individuals in learning to stand up for themselves and live in integrity with their True Self.

Ingredients: Wild Orange, Clove Bud, Cinnamon Bark, Eucalyptus radiate, Rosemary

Suggested Uses: Place 3-5 drops in a capsule and take internally. Inhale regularly throughout the day.

Emotions Addressed: Attacked, Unprotected and Vulnerable, Susceptibility to Peer Pressure

PastTense Blend

The Oil of Relief

dōTERRA's PastTense blend was formulated to relieve headaches. However, it also assists individuals in releasing the stress and emotional tension that may have contributed to or caused their headache.

PastTense synergistically combines the powerful relaxation qualities of nine essential. It teaches the body how to calms down and relax. PastTense also helps individuals release the fears that create tension and pain in the physical body. This combination of oils calm severe stress, soothes trauma, helps prevent nervous breakdowns, and brings balance to the body and energy system. PastTense also helps the individual regain equilibrium following periods of overwork, burnout, and fatigue.

PastTense reminds us to be appreciative. It helps the individual feel gratitude for, and enjoyment in, their many life experiences.

Ingredients: Wintergreen, Lavender, Peppermint, Frankincense, Cilantro, Roman Chamomile, Marjoram, Basil, Rosemary

Suggested Uses: Rub on location of physical pain or discomfort. Inhale regularly throughout the day.

Emotions Addressed: Stress, Overworked, Burnout, Overwhelmed, Breakdown, Nervous, Fatigue

Purify Blend

The Oil of Purification

dōTERRA's Purify blend assists in cleansing and purifying. Purify can assist emotionally toxic individuals to enter a cleansing state. It revitalizes the energy field, washing away negative influences. It offers support to individuals when they are feeling trapped by negative emotions. Purify provides freedom from past habits and patterns as it cleanses the whole system. It is especially helpful in combating toxic emotions such as hate, rage, enmeshment, and negative attachment.

Like Lemongrass, Purify makes a wonderful space cleanser. It can clear negative energy in the household as well as purify the air of odor and harmful microorganisms. Diffused in a healing environment, Purify can assist individuals in "cleaning house" by facilitating an emotional breakthrough. In order to heal, we must receive. But in order to receive, we must release old baggage which blocks the new clean energy of life from entering in. Purify supports individuals in constantly releasing the old so they may be open to the new.

Ingredients: Lemon, Lime, Pine, Citronella, Melaleuca, Cilantro

Suggested Uses: Place 1-2 drops on the heart. Place 10-12 drops in a spray bottle and mist around room or diffuse in air. Inhale regularly throughout the day.

Emotions Addressed: Trapped, Stuck, Toxic Emotions

Serenity Blend

The Oil of Forgiveness

dōTERRA's Serenity blend has a powerful effect on the heart. It calms feelings of hostility, fear, anger, jealousy, rage and resentment. It supports individuals who struggle to forgive others for their hurtful blunders and behaviors. Serenity oil softens the hardened heart. It assists individuals in overcoming their criticisms and judgments of other people. When an individual expects too much from others, Serenity relaxes their perfectionistic expectations. Serenity assists in viewing other people with tenderness and compassion. It teaches that Divine grace is for all, and reminds us that no one is perfect. The need to blame others stems from unhappiness and pain in one's own life. Serenity encourages us to look at our ourselves first when we feel like blaming someone else.

As the individual addresses their own pain, Serenity is very supportive. It brings a person more in touch with the feminine qualities of love, openness and receptivity. Serenity balances the emotional life by healing the wounds in the heart so that love may flow freely. This oil fosters tenderness and love in every relationship. It assists the heart in remaining "whole" by practicing principles of forgiveness.

Ingredients: Lavender, Marjoram, Roman Chamomile, Ylang Ylang, Sandalwood, Vanilla Bean Extract

Suggested Uses: Place 1-3 drops on heart. Inhale regularly throughout the day.

Emotions Addressed: Resentment, Unwillingness to Forgive, Bitterness, Anger, Sadness, Perfectionism

Slim & Sassy Blend

The Oil of Inner Beauty

dōTERRA's Slim & Sassy oil addresses personal patterns of being excessively hard on one's self. These individuals may have an excessive concern for cosmetic grooming. Being overly picky of their physical appearance, they obsess over their imperfections. They set strict standards for themselves in diet or weight loss programs, believing that denying themselves of dietary pleasures will create the desired result. Instead, their punitive withholding is met with whiplash from the body as it desperately seeks to survive. This time, the need for foods/sweets is excessive and out of control. These swings in diet, weight and mood are now met with discouragement as the individual berates their body with self-criticism. There is a hatred and disgust for one's physical body. This personality can also be resistant to the natural aging process, seeking to remain eternally youthful.

Slim & Sassy supports in clearing the heavy emotional weight of self-abuse. It drops pounds of emotional baggage. Slim & Sassy helps an individual to find feelings self-worth. It supports them in loving and accepting their physical body. It encourages them to rise above self-judgments by embracing the body's natural beauty and inherent value, regardless of weight, shape, or size.

Ingredients: Grapefruit, Lemon, Peppermint, Ginger, Cinnamon

Suggested Uses: Place 1-3 drops in a glass of water. Inhale regularly throughout the day.

Emotions Addressed: Self-Criticism, Worthlessness, Feeling Ugly, Disgust/Hate for the Physical Appearance

Solace Blend

The Oil of Vulnerability

dōTERRA's Solace blend encourages warmth in relationships, stabilizes emotional imbalances and fosters emotional intimacy. It is a perfect oil for supporting pregnancy and child delivery, as it strengthens the mother-child bond. It can assist the mother in staying emotionally open so she may connect with her newborn child. Solace is a wonderful oil for mothers. It assists women in accepting their maternal instincts and nurturing qualities.

Solace warms relationships by teaching individuals to be open and vulnerable. It eases one's fears of rejection as one experiences true warmth and love from another person. Solace also encourages feeling empathy for others. It reminds individuals to also stay receptive to the thoughts and feelings of other people.

Solace works as a powerful emotional balancer during menstruation or menopause. It releases emotional tension within the reproductive organs. It releases expectations of suffering and dread related to the monthly cycle. Solace encourages a healthy celebration of one's aging and maturation process.

Ingredients: Clary Sage, Lavender, Bergamot, Roman Chamomile, Cedarwood, Ylang Ylang, Geranium, Fennel, Carrot Seed, Palmarosa, Vitex

Suggested Uses: Place 3-5 drops on abdomen, on heart or over cramping muscles. Inhale regularly throughout the day.

Emotions Addressed: Invulnerability, Guarded, Closed, Dread of Menstruation or Menopause

TerraShield Blend

The Oil of Shielding

dōTERRA's TerraShield blend was formulated as an insect repellent, but offers so much more than that. This blend's protective qualities help an individual stay calm in the face of danger or attack. TerraShield strengthens the protective shield around one's body helping them to feel safe. This is especially important for children and adults who unconsciously "merge" with other people's energy. This may be done as a way to relieve others burdens, or to simply "lighten the load" in the environment. Regardless of the motives, this type of energetic merging weakens an individual's energy system. Babies and young children are especially susceptible to trying to carry loved one's feelings for them, as they struggle to know which emotion's are theirs and which belong to other people. TerraShield assists an individual in separating their own energy from another person's.

While the confusion between boundaries is often unintentional, there are also those who would target or attack another person. This oil teaches individuals to hold strong boundaries and not allow themselves to be pushed around. It imbues individuals with courage and confidence to stand up for themselves and face their attackers.

Ingredients: Lemon, Eucalyptus, Citronella, Lemongrass and a propriety blend of 12 other oils

Suggested Uses: Place 7-10 drops in a spray bottle and mist around body or rub 1-2 drops on wrists and ears. Inhale regularly throughout the day.

Emotions Addressed: Unprotected, Attacked, Defenseless

Whisper Blend

The Oil of Femininity

The dōTERRA Whisper blend is titled "A Blend for Women." However, its benefits are not limited to women alone. While Whisper oil possesses a strong feminine quality, its "female energy" is often needed by both men and women.

Whisper softens the overly-masculine individual by getting them in touch with their feminine side. It encourages individuals to let go of pride and let down their "tough" exterior. When placed over the liver, Whisper can ease feelings of anger. It calms tension, irritability and malice. Whisper encourages adaptability.

Whisper's feminine nature assists individuals in healing relationships with mothers, grandmothers and other women. It helps us to reconnect to our mother when there has been strain, separation, loss, or abuse in the relationship. It challenges us to work through our issues relating to both femininity as well as sexuality. If we have rejected our own female side, Whisper invites us to heal our wounds and bring balance to our female energies.

Ingredients: Patchouli, Bergamot, Sandalwood, Rose, Jasmine, Cinnamon Bark, Cistus, Vetiver, Ylang Ylang, Geranium, Cocoa Bean Extract, Vanilla Bean Extract

Suggested Uses: Place 1-3 drops over the womb or just below the naval. Inhale regularly throughout the day.

Emotions Addressed: Overly Masculine, Unteachable, Strain in Feminine Energies, Anger, Irritable

Zendocrine Blend

The Oil of Transition

dōTERRA's Zendocrine blend was formulated to cleanse the organs of the body. Emotionally, Zendocrine assists during times of transition and change. It assists individuals in "detoxing" old habits and limiting beliefs. When an individual has felt trapped by self-sabotaging behaviors or addictions, Zendocrine paves the way for new life experiences. It aids us in letting go of behaviors that are destructive to our health and happiness. It is especially helpful during major life changes which require adjustments in habit and lifestyle such as: altering diet, quitting smoking, or leaving a toxic relationship. Zendocrine is a great aid in these times of major transition.

The oils in this blend encourage us to let go of the non-essentials or anything that sabotages our higher purpose. Zendocrine provides inner strength to make these commitments and follow through with them. As we let go of self-limiting beliefs, behaviors and lifestyles, we have greater room to receive. As a result, we are able to see life with a fresh perspective.

Ingredients: Clove, Grapefruit, Rosemary, Geranium

Suggested Uses: Place 3-5 drops in capsule and take internally. Inhale regularly throughout the day.

Emotions Addressed: Difficulty with Transitions

Section III

Appendices

Appendix A

Application Through
Muscle Testing

Muscle Response Testing is a quick and simple way in which we can access information from the body/subconscious for our healing. It allows us to bypass the conscious mind by tapping into a deeper source of wisdom and information.

How to Learn Muscle Testing

Those interested in learning how to Muscle Test may visit our website at: **www.discovertruthwithin.com** to obtain a series of 4-DVD's which teach in full detail how to muscle test for yourself and those you work with.

Testing for Specific Oils

Use the lists at the end of Appendix A to test which oil(s) you need. First test the number of oils you will be using, then test each one to determine whether it is a single or blend. Once you have identified your oils you may then test for application.

Testing for Application

dōTERRA Essential oils can be used in three ways.

You may want to test one or more ways the oil should be used:

1. Aromatic
2. Internal (dōTERRA only!)
3. Topical

**As you test, you will need to reference safety information in *Modern Essentials* to know which oils are safe for internal use, children, pregnancy, etc., and which are not.

Aromatic

If the oil is for aromatic use, you either smell it regularly from the bottle, or place a few drops in a diffuser.

Internal

If the oil is for internal use, check the safety information to ensure that it is safe. If you are taking an essential oil that is irritating to the skin or throat, put the drops into a capsule. If you test for a large quantity of oil, use a capsule.

**Note: do not mix different oils in the same capsule unless you are certain they "blend" well together. Test the number of drops you need. Also test how many times a day you need to take the oil.

Sample testing questions:

Testing number of drops: "I need one or more drops of [essential oil (i.e. lemon oil)]."

Testing how many times a day you need the drops: "I need [however many drops you tested] once a day." Then continue testing, "twice a day," "three times a day," and so on.

Topical

If the oil is for topical use, test whether the oil should be applied diluted or "neat" (undiluted) on skin. Also test the part(s) of the body the oil should be applied to. Then go back to the steps above and test the quantity and regularity.

Possible parts of the body for application:

1. Arms
2. Ears
3. Face
4. Feet
5. Hands
6. Heart
7. Legs
8. Neck/Throat
9. Shoulders
10. Spine
12. Stomach

*When using more than one oil, layer them one by one.

dōTERRA SINGLE OILS TESTING LIST

1. Basil
2. Bergamot
3. Birch
4. Cassia
5. Cinnamon
6. Clary Sage
7. Clove Bud
8. Coriander
9. Cypress
10. Eucalyptus
11. Fennel
12. Frankincense
13. Geranium
14. Ginger
15. Grapefruit
16. Helichrysum
17. Lavender
18. Lemon
19. Lemongrass
20. Lime
21. Marjoram
22. Melaleuca
23. Melissa
24. Myrrh
25. Orange, Wild
26. Oregano
27. Patchouli
28. Peppermint
29. Roman Chamomile
30. Rose
31. Rosemary
32. Sandalwood
33. Thyme
34. Vetiver
35. White Fir
36. Wintergreen
37. Ylang Ylang

dōTERRA OIL BLENDS TESTING LIST

1. AromaTouch
2. Balance
3. Breathe
4. Citrus Bliss
5. Clear Skin Topical Blend
6. Deep Blue
7. DigestZen
8. Elevation
9. OnGuard
10. PastTense
11. Purify
12. Serenity
13. Slim & Sassy
14. Solace
15. TerraShield
16. Whisper

Appendix B

Essential Oils for Addiction

Oils Recommended for Addiction in General

- Bergamot
- Frankincense
- Peppermint
- Vetiver
- White Fir
- Zendocrine

Bergamot

Bergamot is recommended for all addictions because of its ability to move an individual out of self-judgment. Addiction recovery is almost always accompanied by bouts of relapse. When this happens, an individual will often beat themselves up for days or weeks. These feelings of self-beat up are not helpful in addiction recovery. In fact, they can throw the individual more deeply into their addictive patterns or addictive cycle. Bergamot can assist the individual in maintaining unconditional self-love and acceptance. While accepting one's self and one's addiction may be the most difficult thing to do, it is also the most healing step. When an individual does not fear their own judgment for making mistakes, they are more likely to succeed. Bergamot is therefore a suggested staple in any addiction recovery.

Frankincense

Frankincense is highly recommended in all addictions for its ability to rid the body of darkness and negativity, and assist the individual in seeing truth.

Peppermint

Peppermint is recommended for periodic use in all cases of addiction. Peppermint brings buoyancy and joy to the soul. When the path feels too difficult for one to bear, Peppermint can bring relief from the intense pain felt in the heart and mind. <u>Peppermint should not be used as an escape to one's problems, but rather as a periodic support during times of extreme heaviness and when one feels hopelessness and or despair.</u> Peppermint can help an individual re-discover joy in living and hope for healing.

Vetiver

Vetiver is recommended for in addictions for addressing the underlying emotional issue of the addiction. Vetiver assists an individual in uncovering the "root" of an emotional issue. It connects the person deeply with the Self and whatever is truly going on inside. Vetiver can assist the individual in facing the issue head on instead of running away from their pain through some sort of escape/addiction.

White Fir

White Fir is recommended for all addictions that are "generational" in nature. This means that the addiction has been passed down by one or more family members. Perhaps a parent, grandparent, sibling, or other relative shares a similar addiction. In such cases, White Fir can assist in breaking these negative generational patterns so the entire family can "come clean." Note: most all addictions have a "generational" root.

Zendocrine

Zendocrine is recommended for many kinds of addiction. It assists an individual in letting go of what no longer serves them. Zendocrine is a great aid in times of transition and change. It is especially helpful in making life changes which require adjustments in habit or lifestyle, such as a change of diet, quitting smoking, or leaving a toxic relationship.

Additional Support

*Supporting the glands of the brain as well as the liver can be helpful in all kinds of addiction recovery. For brain support (hippocampus, thalamus, hypothalamus, pineal and pituitary) place a few drops of Sandalwood, Frankincense or Immortelle across the brow. To support the liver, apply Lemongrass, Cypress, Helichrysum, Geranium or Grapefruit over the liver.

Oils Recommended for Specific Addictions

CAFFINE/ENERGY DRINKS

- Basil
- Slim & Sassy

Basil

When a person feels burned-out, they are more likely to seek stimulants that give pseudo energy to the body, or a false pick-me-up for the mind. Basil oil assists an individual in giving up all kinds of substance addiction linked to the physical body. It assists in clearing negative thinking patterns, releasing toxic energies and renewing the physical body. Basil assists the body in finding natural sources of energy available when one follows its natural rhythms and laws of health. This oil is indicated for those who are weary in mind and body and who need energy and strength. (Place 5-10 drops+ or so on bottoms of feet and inhale from the bottle regularly throughout the day.)

Slim & Sassy

Slim & Sassy assists an individual in listening to their physical body. It stimulates a natural sense of energy in the body which stems from balance and health. (Place a few drops in glass of water and drink throughout the day.)

DRUGS & ALCOHOL

- Basil
- Zendocrine
- Frankincense
- Roman Chamomile

Basil

Basil oil assists an individual in giving up addictions to substances. It assists in clearing negative thinking patterns, releasing toxic energies and renewing the physical body. (Place 5-6+ drops on bottom of feet and over liver as well as inhale from the bottle throughout the day)

Zendocrine

Zendocrine has a powerful ability to remove toxins from the physical body. It is also indicated for drug and alcohol addictions for its ability to assist an individual in letting go of what no longer serves them emotionally. It is a great aid in times of transition and change. It is especially helpful in making life changes which require adjustments in habit or lifestyle, such as coming off drugs. (Place 5-6+ drops on bottom of feet or over any organ or gland in need of assistance. Also inhale from the bottle regularly throughout the day.)

Frankincense

Frankincense clears the intense forms of darkness and negativity often associated with drug abuse. It also assists a person in feeling the love and protection from a Higher Power. Frankincense challenges a person to leave behind negativity and lies and align with truth. (Place a few drops under the tongue each day and inhale from the bottle regularly.)

Roman Chamomile

Roman Chamomile assists an individual in living true to the self by making choices aligned with one's spiritual purpose. It helps a person to see when their patterns or lifestyle choices are not in harmony with their greatest good. Our true nature blossoms gradually under the warmth of the sun. Like a guardian angel, Chamomile leads an individual to where they need to be and what they need to be doing. It removes distractions and helps them to focus on fulfilling their true purpose. (Place a few drops over the solar plexus or upper stomach and inhale regularly from bottle throughout the day.)

Additional Support

*Oils that support/cleanse the liver are also recommended for drug and alcohol addictions: Lemongrass, Geranium, Helichrysum, Cypress, or Grapefruit. (Apply oils over liver)

EATING DISORDERS, Anorexia/Bulimia

- Grapefruit
- Slim & Sassy
- Bergamot
- Cinnamon

Grapefruit

Assists an individual in honoring the physical body. Grapefruit encourages a person to "listen" to the needs and impulses of the body, such as hunger, the need to eat or when the body is satiated/full. (Inhale from bottle regularly and place a few drops over heart.)

Slim & Sassy

Assists the individual in addressing deep feelings of shame and unworthiness which is often a root cause of anorexia and bulimia. This oil should not be used internally in large quantities in cases of anorexia or bulimia, but should instead be diffused or used in small quantities for its emotional benefits. (Place a drop or two over the heart and inhale regularly from bottle.)

Bergamot

Bergamot can assist the individual in learning to love and accept the self unconditionally. This need to love one's self lies at the heart of anorexia and bulimia. (Place a drop under the tongue each day and inhale from the bottle throughout the day.)

Cinnamon

Helps an individual to accept their body as it is by seeing its natural beauty. (Place a few drops on the feet. You may need to mix the cinnamon with fractionated coconut oil if you have sensitive skin. Also inhale from the bottle regularly throughout the day.)

EATING DISORDERS, Foods/Over-eating
(chocolate, sugar, fatty foods, etc)

- Grapefruit
- Basil
- Thyme
- Slim & Sassy

Grapefruit

Grapefruit is one of the finest oils for curbing emotional eating. It brings to conscious awareness our relationship with food and the physical body. It assists us in taking more responsibility for not only what we eat but also what we feel. It teaches that no amount of food can fill the holes in our hearts, only love can do that. As we take ownership of what we feel, and address our upset feelings, we no longer have a need to hide our feelings behind food. (Place a few drops in a glass of water and drink throughout the day)

Basil

Assists an individual in listening to the natural rhythms of the body, including the natural impulses to rest, to sleep or to stop eating. (Place a few drops on the bottom of the feet and inhale from the bottle regularly)

Thyme

Thyme powerfully cleanses emotional issues from the heart. It is especially helpful in addressing feelings of anger and resentment often associated with overeating. Thyme counters the need to "stuff" or "eat" feelings such as sadness, anger, or disappointment. Thyme can open the heart and assist in facing all kinds of negative emotions. (Place a few drops in empty capsule and take internally)

Slim & Sassy

Slim & Sassy assists an individual in listening to their physical body. It addresses deep feelings of shame and unworthiness that often associated with overeating. It also assists individuals in curbing emotional eating, balancing blood sugar, and losing weight. (Place a few drops in a glass of water and drink throughout the day.)

ENTERTAINMENT (computers, internet, shopping, television, videogames, etc.)

- Vetiver
- Serenity
- Balance

Vetiver

Vetiver assists an individual in uncovering the "root" of an emotional issue. The need for entertainment acts as an escape from pain and dis-satisfaction with one's life. Vetiver connects a person with their life and whatever is going on inside. In this way, it assists a person in addressing the real issue head on, instead of running away from the pain through escapism. (Place a few drops on temples, over brow or on stomach. Also inhale from bottle regularly throughout the day.)

Serenity

Serenity calms and stabilizes one's emotions. It can assist an individual in addressing deep emotional issues as well as calm fear and anxieties. (Place a few drops over stomach, inhale regularly from bottle throughout day.)

Balance

Balance assists an individual in creating balance and moderation in each aspect of life. It is also "grounding," assisting an individual to face the reality of their life's situation. (Place a few drops on bottom of feet and inhale from bottle regularly throughout the day.)

PORNOGRAPHY

- Frankincense
- Helichrysum

Frankincense

Frankincense clears the intense forms of darkness and negativity that comes with Pornography. It also assists individuals in being honest with themselves and other people. Frankincense challenges a person to leave behind negativity and lies by aligning with truth. (Place a few drops under the tongue each day and inhale from the bottle regularly.)

Helichrysum

Helichrysum contacts the energy of new life and rebirth. It lends its warrior spirit so that an individual may face their trials with courage, determination and honesty. Helichrysum takes the wounded soul by the hand guiding them through life's difficulties. (Place a single drop over solar plexus. Inhale from bottle regularly throughout the day.)

SELF-INJURY

- Oregano
- Frankincense

Oregano

Oregano assists an individual in clearing from their lives all that is not truly serving them. This oil powerfully clears negative ties and relationships. It is helpful in clearing out anything that is holding us back in life. Oregano may encourage an individual to leave behind an old friend, oppressive job, or anything that is dragging them down and causing unneeded baggage. (Place a 6-12+ drops into an empty capsule and take internally.)

Frankincense

Frankincense clears the intense forms of darkness and negativity associated with the desire to injure one's self. It can assist the individual in feeling connected to a loving Higher Power. Frankincense challenges a person to leave behind their negative patterns and behaviors by aligning with truth. (Place a few drops under the tongue each day and inhale from the bottle regularly.)

SEXUAL ADDICTION

- Cinnamon
- Purify
- Geranium
- Sandalwood

Cinnamon

Cinnamon assists an individual in balancing sexual energies. It can support when there is either repressed or overactive sexual forces. Cinnamon clears feelings of jealousy and the need to control one's partner. It also assists in allowing one's partner to be free in the relationship rather than being controlled. (Inhale from the bottle regularly throughout the day)

Purify

Purify cleanses the emotional pain and negativity associated with situations of sexual addiction. It assists in clearing negative belief systems such as feeling "unlovable," "unworthy," or "unacceptable." (Place a few drops below the naval and over kidneys. Also Inhale from bottle regularly throughout the day)

Geranium

Geranium supports the heart in feeling unconditional love from the self and others so that one does not need to seek false forms of love. The desperate "need" for sex stems from a lack of feeling unconditional love and true connections in relationships. (Place a few drops over the heart and inhale regularly from the bottle throughout the day)

Sandalwood

Sandalwood supports an individual in feeling connected to Divine love so they do not feel the need to seek false forms of love through sexual pleasure. (Place a few drops on brow and inhale regularly throughout the day.)

TOBACCO

- Clove
- Basil
- Zendocrine

Clove

Clove is indicated for quitting smoking for its ability to cleanse the body and heal the brain, and remove the strong taste of tobacco from the mouth. Individuals quitting smoking or chewing often need something in their mouth, especially to remove the "taste" of tobacco which make the cravings worse. OnGuard lozenges (which have clove oil in them) may be helpful for combating both the taste of, and cravings for tobacco. (May also place a few drops in an empty capsule and take-internally, or place a few drops on toothbrush and brush teeth with the Clove oil or OnGuard oil or toothpaste.)

Basil

Basil oil assists an individual in giving up substance related addictions. It assists in clearing negative thinking patterns, releasing toxic energies and renewing the physical body. (Place a few drops on bottom of feet and inhale regularly from the bottle throughout the day.)

Zendocrine

Zendocrine assists an individual in letting go of what no longer serves them. It is a great aid in times of transition and change. It is especially helpful in making life changes which require adjustments in habit or lifestyle, such as quitting smoking. (Place a few drops in empty capsule and take internally.)

WORK

- Wild Orange
- Ylang Ylang
- Serenity

Wild Orange

Wild Orange supports right brain function and assists an individual in creative thought and expression. Orange helps the person to embrace their fun/creative side. It brings new life and energy and can support the person who tends to be over serious and works long hours. Wild Orange teaches the individual how to relax, laugh more, and enjoy life. Orange brings a powerful sense of trust in the abundance of life and the universe. (Place a few drops below the naval, diffuse in work environment, and inhale directly from bottle throughout the day.)

Ylang Ylang

Ylang Ylang assists an individual in opening the heart, trusting in life, and connecting to their "inner child." It assists the individual in calming nervousness and fear. It supports in opening to feeling life and re-experiencing the ability to have childlike fun. (Place a few drops on heart and inhale regularly from bottle throughout the day.)

Serenity

Serenity brings balance and calm to the individual who is too anxious or "high strung." Serenity calms the whole system. It supports an individual to not worry so much about the necessities of life. Serenity assists in stilling the mind and being present with what is. (Place a few drops over the heart. Inhale regularly from the bottle throughout the day.)

Additional Notes on Addiction:

There are many ways to use the essential oils listed above in addition to what is mentioned here. This appendix contains only a few minor suggestions. For example, applying oils on the ears can be helpful in creating emotional balance and in relieving addictive energy. One technique is to simply apply a drop or two of an essential oil on the wrists, rub them together and then rub the wrists against the ears. A study of auricular therapy could reveal more specific regions the oils may be applied to support a variety of issues.

It is also the author's opinion that any successful recovery program must acknowledge the use of a Higher Power. The essential oils are not a "fix" to addiction. Rather, the oils may be seen as a "support" to other programs and therapies. Time has shown that support groups who encourage individuals to acknowledge a Higher Power are the most effective in addiction recovery. Recognizing one's powerlessness to "will" their way out of an addiction can propel an individual forward in relying on a power greater than one's self. Essential oils are not a substitute to the healing power that comes from the Divine. Oils are a means of accessing states of humility and surrender so that true healing may be accessed.

It is also important to mention here that this reference list is intended as an informational guide. The information contained in this appendix is simply a recommendation. It is in no way intended to substitute for the help of qualified licensed medical or mental health professionals. This appendix is not to be used to make any kind of diagnosis. For a diagnosis, treatment, and recovery program please consult a qualified licensed medical or mental health care professional.

Appendix C

Essential Oil
Emotional Usage Guide

A

Abandoned: Frankincense, Geranium

Abuse: Cinnamon, Clove, Helichrysum, White Fir

Addiction: (see appendix on addiction)

Adjustment, difficulty with: Rosemary, Zendocrine

Afraid: (see Fear)

Agitated: Lavender

Agony: Helichrysum, Clear Skin Blend

Aggression: (see Anger)

Aimless: Roman Chamomile

Alienated: Birch, Myrrh

Aloof: Marjoram, Balance Blend

Anger: Thyme, Serenity Blend, Geranium, Ylang Ylang, Whisper Blend, Clear Skin Blend

Anguish: Helichrysum, Immortelle Blend, Clear Skin Blend

Annoyed: Vetiver, Serenity Blend

Anxious/Anxiety: Basil, Breathe Blend, PastTense Blend

Apathy/Apathetic: Lemongrass, Vetiver, Lime

Appearance, anxiety over: Slim & Sassy Blend, Grapefruit, Clear Skin Blend

Appearance, negative image of: Slim & Sassy Blend, Grapefruit, Clear Skin Blend

Appetite, loss of: DigestZen Blend, Fennel

Apprehensive: Cassia, Cinnamon, Melissa

Argumentative: Lavender

Arrogant: Whisper Blend, Solace

Ashamed: (see Shame)

Assimilate, inability to: DigestZen Blend, Wild Orange, Rosemary

Attached, overly: Oregano, Sandalwood

Attacked: OnGuard Blend, Terrashield Blend, Birch

Avoidance: Deep Blue Blend, Vetiver, Balance Blend

B

Bad (as in feeling that "I am bad"): Bergamot, Slim & Sassy Blend

Baffled: (see Confusion)

Barriers, emotional: Marjoram, Solace Blend, Serenity Blend, Cassia

Bashful: Cassia, Cinnamon, Ginger

Beaten Down: OnGuard Blend

Belittled: Bergamot, Slim & Sassy

Betrayed: (see Cheated)

Bewildered: (see Confused)

Bitterness: Serenity Blend, Thyme

Blah: (see Apathy)

Blaming: Clear Skin Blend, Serenity Blend, Vetiver, Ginger

Blindness, spiritual: Immortelle Blend, Clary Sage, Lemongrass

Blocked, emotionally: Cypress, Thyme, Peppermint, Oregano

Boastful: (see Pride)

Body, disconnection from: Balance, Patchouli, Vetiver

Body, hate for: Grapefruit, Slim & Sassy Blend

Body, judgment of: Grapefruit, Slim & Sassy Blend, Patchouli

Body, rejection of: Cinnamon, Slim & Sassy Blend

Body shame: Patchouli

Body tension: PastTense Blend, AromaTouch Blend, Patchouli

Bondage, emotional: Thyme, Zendocrine Blend

Boundaries, poor: OnGuard Blend, Melaleuca, Clove, TerraShield Blend, Oregano

Bragging: (see Pride)

Breakdown: PastTense Blend, Peppermint

Breath, constricted: Breathe Blend, AromaTouch Blend, Peppermint, White Fir

Burdened: White Fir, Wintergreen

Burned out: Basil, PastTense Blend, Breathe Blend

C

Captive: (see Bondage, Emotional)

Careless: (see Apathy/Apathetic)

Chaos/Chaotic: Lemon, Vetiver

Cheated: (see Betrayed)

Clingy: Eucalyptus, Ylang Ylang

Closed, emotionally: Ylang Ylang, Solace Blend

Closed-minded: Wild Orange, Rosemary

Co-dependent: Melaleuca, Clove, OnGuard

Cold: (see Aloof)

Communication, blocked: Lavender, Whisper Blend

Competitive: Whisper Blend, Helichrysum

Complaining: Elevation Blend, Ylang Ylang

Compulsive: Sandalwood

Conceited: Whisper, Solace Blend

Condemning: (see Judgmental)

Confined: (see Trapped)

Conforming: Coriander, Clove, Ginger, Cassia

Confused/Confusion: Clary Sage, Lemon, Peppermint, Rosemary

Constricted: Lavender, Cypress

Contentious: Serenity Blend

Controlling /Control, need to: Cinnamon, Wintergreen, Cypress

Controlled: OnGuard Blend, Clove, Coriander

Cowardly: Clove, Cassia, Cinnamon

Cranky: Whisper, Serenity Blend

Creativity, blocked or stifled: Citrus Bliss Blend, Wild Orange, Clary Sage

Critical: Bergamot, Slim & Sassy Blend, Clear Skin Blend

Criticized: Bergamot

Crying: (see Sadness)

Cursed: Melissa

Cynical: Wild Orange, Clear Skin Blend

D

Dark, in the: Immortelle Blend, Melissa, Clary Sage, Elevation Blend

Darkness: Lemongrass, Frankincense, Immortelle Blend

Death, acceptance of: Roman Chamomile, Frankincense, Cypress

Death Wish: (see Suicidal)

Deceived: Clary Sage

Defeated: Clove, Citrus Bliss Blend, Eucalyptus, Ginger, Fennel

Defenseless: TerraShield Blend, OnGaurd Blend

Defensive: Whisper Blend, Solace Blend, Ylang Ylang, Geranium

Defiant: Whisper Blend, Ylang Ylang,

Defiled: Purify Blend, Thyme

Degraded: Bergamot, Clove

Denial: Clary Sage, Thyme, Deep Blue Blend, Vetiver, Immortelle Blend

Dependent: Melaleuca, Clove

Depressed/Depression: Elevation Blend, Peppermint, Melissa, Citrus Bliss Blend

Desire, lack of: Balance Blend, Fennel

Despair: Bergamot, Eucalyptus, Lemongrass

Despondent: Melissa, Eucalyptus, Balance Blend

Dieting, addiction to: (See section on addiction)

Dirty: Purify Blend, Zendocrine Blend, Patchouli

Disassociation from Body: Balance Blend, Vetiver, Myrrh

Disconnected: Balance Blend, Vetiver, Marjoram

Disconnected from Body: Patchouli

Disconnection, spiritual: Frankincense, Sandalwood, Clary Sage

Discontent: Wild Orange, Clear Skin Blend

Discouraged: Lime, Wild Orange, Clary Sage, Roman Chamomile

Disgust/Disgusting: Slim & Sassy Blend

Disharmony: Balance Blend, Serenity Blend

Disheartened: Rose, Geranium

Dishonest: Clary Sage, Frankincense, Ginger

Distant: Marjoram

Distressed: Immortelle Blend

Distrusting: Geranium, Marjoram, Myrrh

Divided/Double Minded: Balance Blend, Vetiver

Dominated: Clove, OnGuard Blend, TerraShield Blend

Doubtful: Sandalwood

Drained: Basil, PastTense Blend, AromaTouch Blend

Dread: Fennel, Solace Blend

Dreary: Melissa

Drudgery: Fennel, Coriander, Roman Chamomile

Dull: Citrus Bliss Blend, Wild Orange

Dumb: Lemon, Peppermint, Rosemary

E

Egotistical/Egotism: Whisper Blend

Embarrassed: Cassia

Emptiness: Vetiver, Sandalwood

Energy, lack of: Lemon, Peppermint, Wild Orange, Elevation Blend, Citrus Bliss Blend

Enslaved: Clove, Thyme, Fennel

Entangled: Melaleuca, Clove, OnGuard Blend

Escape: Eucalyptus

Exasperated: Basil, Breathe Blend, Lavender

Excessive: Balance Blend, Sandalwood

Exhausted: Basil

F

Façade, emotional: Vetiver, Deep Blue Blend, Helichrysum, Zendocrine Blend, Purify Blend

Failure (as in "I am a failure"): Bergamot, Roman Chamomile

Faithless: Sandalwood

Father, distant from: Frankincense

Fatigued: Basil, Breathe Blend, PastTense Blend

Fatigued, mental: Lemon, Breathe Blend

Fear/Fearful: Cassia, Cinnamon, Birch, Cypress

Feminine Energy, imbalance of: Whisper Blend

Filthy (see Dirty)

Flighty: Balance Blend

Floundering: Balance Blend, Lemon

Focus, inability to: Lemon, Peppermint

Food, addiction to: Grapefruit, Slim & Sassy

Foolish: Cassia

Forgetful: Lemon, Peppermint

Fragmented: Vetiver, Balance Blend

Frantic: Breathe Blend, PastTense Blend

Friendless: Marjoram, Geranium

Frustrated: Geranium, Roman Chamomile

Furious: Geranium, Rose

G

Generational Issues: White Fir, Birch

Giving up: Helichrysum, Deep Blue Blend

Gloomy: Deep Blue Blend

Greedy: Wild Orange

Grief: Deep Blue Blend, Geranium

Grouchy: Whisper, Thyme

Guarded: Solace Blend

Guilt: Bergamot, Lemon, Peppermint

Gullible: Clary Sage

H

Harassed: OnGuard Blend, TerraShield Blend

Hardened: Rose, Geranium, Serenity Blend

Hard-Hearted: Rose, Geranium, Serenity Blend, Thyme

Harsh: Marjoram

Hasty: (see Impatience)

Hate/Hateful/Hatred: Thyme

Haughty: (see also Egotistical)

Haunted: Frankincense, OnGuard Blend

Headstrong: Wild Orange, Whisper Blend, Lime

Heartbroken: Geranium

Heartless: Rose, Geranium

Heavy-Hearted: Lime, Elevation, Geranium

Helpless/Helplessness: Clove, Ginger, OnGuard

Hereditary Issues: (see Generational Issues)

Hiding: Cassia

Holding onto the past: Thyme, Lemongrass, Purify, Zendocrine

Hoarding: Lemongrass, Myrrh

Hopeless: Clary Sage, Immortelle Blend

Humiliated: Cassia

Hurried: Breathe Blend, PastTense Blend

Hurtful to others: Whisper, Serenity, Rose

Hypocritical: Clary Sage, Frankincense

Hysterical: Breathe Blend, Balance, Deep Blue Blend

I

Ignorant: Rosemary

Illness, attached to: Eucalyptus

Imbalanced, emotionally: Serenity Blend, Citrus Bliss Blend

Immobilized: Cypress, Thyme

Immoral: Frankincense, Zendocrine Blend, Purify Blend

Impatient/Impatience: (see Aggression, Agitated, Anger, Anxiety)

Impoverished: Wild Orange

Imprisoned: Eucalyptus, Lavender, Zendocrine

Inadequate: Bergamot, Slim & Sassy Blend, Clear Skin Blend

Incapable: Bergamot

Inconsiderate of others: Cinnamon, Serenity Blend

Inconsistent: Coriander, Balance Blend

Indecisive: Lemon, Peppermint

Indifferent: (see Apathy)

Inferior: Bergamot

Inflexible: AromaTouch Blend

Insecure: Cassia

Insight, lack of: Immortelle Blend, Clary Sage, Frankincense

Insignificant: Slim & Sassy Blend

Instability: Balance Blend

Intimidated: Clove

Intolerant: Geranium, Rose, Clear Skin Blend

Introvert: Marjoram

Invulnerable: Solace Blend, Marjoram

Irritated: Whisper Blend, Serenity Blend, Solace Blend

Irresponsible: Fennel, Ginger, Balance Blend

Isolated: Marjoram, Myrrh

J

Jealousy: Cinnamon

Joy, lack of: Elevation, Lemon, Ylang Ylang

Judged: Birch, Clove, Ginger, Cassia

Judgmental: Whisper, Geranium, Rose, Ylang Ylang

K

Know it all: Oregano, Whisper, Rosemary, Wintergreen

L

Learning Disorders: Lemon, Rosemary, DigestZen

Left out: Marjoram, Myrrh

Less than: Bergamot, Clear Skin Blend

Limited thinking: Oregano, Rosemary, Coriander, DigestZen

Loathsome: Slim & Sassy Blend, Patchouli

Loneliness: Marjoram, Frankincense, Myrrh

Loss: Geranium, Ylang Ylang

Lost/Purposeless: Roman Chamomile, Frankincense

Low Self-Esteem/Self-Worth: Bergamot

Lustful: Cinnamon

M

Mad: (see Anger)

Malnourished: Myrrh, DigestZen

Manipulated: Clove

Manipulative: Cinnamon, Solace Blend

Masculine, overly: Whisper Blend, Solace Blend

Materialistic: Sandalwood, Oregano

Maternal Connection, disrupted: Myrrh, Solace Blend, Whisper Blend

Mean: Geranium, Ylang Ylang, Whisper

Menopause, dread of: Solace Blend

Menstruation, dread of: Solace Blend

Melancholy: (see Sadness)

Moody/Unstable Moods: Elevation Blend, Wild Orange

Muddled: Peppermint

N

Narrow-minded: Rosemary, Oregano, Wild Orange, Lemon

Need for approval: Bergamot

Negative Energy: Lemongrass, Melaleuca, Thyme, Oregano, Purify Blend

Neglected: Solace Blend, Myrrh

Nervousness: Basil, Wild Orange, PastTense Blend

Not enough: (see Scarcity)

Numb: (see Apathy)

O

Obsessed: Patchouli

Obsessive-compulsive: Sandalwood, Bergamot, Purify

Obstinate: Whisper Blend

Offended: Serenity, Geranium

Opinionated: Oregano

Oppressed: Clove, OnGuard, White Fir

Out of control: Balance Blend

Outraged: (see Anger)

Over-analyzing: Wild Orange, Ylang Ylang

Over-Empathetic: (see Boundaries)

Overloaded: Thyme

Over-thinking: Sandalwood, Myrrh, Ylang Ylang, Wild Orange

Overwhelmed: Basil, AromaTouch Blend, PastTense Blend

Overworked: Wild Orange, Ylang Ylang, PastTense Blend

Overly-sensitive: TerraShield, OnGuard, Clove, Ginger

P

Pain, emotional: Helichrysum, Deep Blue Blend

Pain, resistance to: Deep Blue Blend, Helichrysum

Paranoia: Vetiver, Breathe Blend

Peer pressure, susceptible to: Ginger, Clove, OnGuard

Perfectionism: Cypress, Serenity Blend

Persecuted: OnGuard

Pessimistic: Basil, Peppermint

Poor, financially: Wild Orange

Possessive: Sandalwood, Oregano

Poverty-stricken: (see Poor)

Powerless: Clove, Ginger

Powerless to heal: Eucalyptus

Prejudice: Oregano

Protected: Marjoram, Serenity Blend, Geranium

Procrastination: Ginger

Proud: Oregano, Whisper Blend

Punishing: Slim & Sassy Blend

Purposeless: Roman Chamomile

Q

Quarrelsome: Whisper, Oregano

Quick-tempered: Geranium, Solace Blend

Quitting: Helichrysum

R

Rage: Thyme

Reclusive: Marjoram

Rejection, fear of: Lavender, Cinnamon

Relationships, co-dependent: Melaleuca, Clove, OnGuard Blend

Relationships, parasitic: Melaleuca, OnGuard, Oregano

Resentment: Serenity Blend, Geranium, Thyme

Resignation: Lime

Resistance: Vetiver, Deep Blue Blend, DigestZen Blend

Responsibility: Fennel, Ginger, Balance Blend, Grapefruit

Rigid: Cypress, Oregano, Wild Orange

S

Sadness: Serenity Blend, Ylang Ylang, Peppermint

Scarcity: Wild Orange

Scattered: Vetiver

Self-betrayal: Coriander

Self-criticism: Slim & Sassy Blend, Bergamot

Self-expression, fear of: Citrus Bliss Blend, Lavender

Self-expression, blocked: Lavender

Self-judgment: Bergamot

Self-Sabotage: Slim & Sassy

Self, weak sense of: Vetiver, Ginger, Balance Blend, Fennel

Serious, overly: Citrus Bliss Blend, Elevation Blend, Wild Orange

Sexually Imbalanced: Cinnamon, Whisper Blend

Sexual Identity, acceptance of: Cinnamon

Sexual repression: Cinnamon

Shame: Balance Blend, Fennel

Shame, body: Patchouli

Shy: Cassia

Sickly: Eucalyptus

Soul, dark night of: Immortelle Blend

Split: Vetiver

Stern: Elevation Blend, Wild Orange, Citrus Bliss Blend, Whisper Blend

Stiffness (body or mind): AromaTouch Blend

Stressed: AromaTouch Blend, Vetiver, Ylang Ylang, PastTense Blend

Stuck: Cypress, Purify Blend

Suicidal: Citrus Bliss Blend, Melissa, Immortelle Blend, Frankincense, Lime

T

Tense: AromaTouch Blend, PastTense Blend, Cypress

Tension, body: AromaTouch Blend, PastTense Blend, Cypress, Patchouli

Tired: Basil

Toxic energy: Lemongrass, Melaleuca, Purify Blend

Toxicity: Melaleuca, Purify Blend, Zendocrine

Transitioning, difficulty with: Rosemary, Zendocrine Blend

Trapped: Thyme, Clary Sage, Purify Blend, Zendocrine Blend

Turmoil: Helichrysum

U

Ugly: Slim & Sassy, Clear Skin Blend

Unforgiving: Serenity Blend, Rose, Geranium, Thyme

Unheard: Lavender

Unlovable: Bergamot

Unloving: Geranium, Rose, Serenity Blend

Unprotected: OnGuard Blend, TerraShield Blend

Unsafe in the world: Myrrh, OnGuard Blend

Unseen: Lavender

Unsettled: Roman Chamomile

Unsupported: Birch, Frankincense

Unteachable: Rosemary, Whisper Blend

V

Victim: Clove, Ginger

Violated: OnGuard Blend

Violent: Serenity Blend

Vulnerable: OnGuard Blend, TerraShield Blend

W

Weak-willed: Birch, Melaleuca, Ginger, Clove, Wintergreen

Weary: Basil

Workaholic: Wild Orange, Ylang Ylang

Willful, excessively: Oregano, Wintergreen

Worried: Breathe Blend

Wounded: Helichrysum

Worthless: Cassia, Bergamot, Slim & Sassy Blend

Appendix D

Enlighten

Enlighten, LLC is composed of four founding partners:

Amanda Porter
Chuck Call
Daniel Macdonald
Sarah McCann

Each partner strives to promote overall
health and wellness through providing
quality materials, services, and healing opportunities.

About Enlighten

Enlighten assists individuals in transformative healing and in discovering their true, authentic selves. We believe healing comes from the inside-out and originates in our relationship with the Divine. Our mission is to enlighten souls through truth by offering quality products and healing services.

Emotional Education

If you would like to learn more about
emotional and spiritual healing, please visit our website at:

www.discovertruthwithin.com